unleash
— the —
THIN
within

the spirit, mind, and body solution
to permanent weight loss

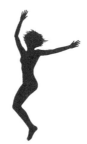

MARGIANNA LANGSTON

HBS
strategies
Decatur, GA

HBS Strategies Inc.
3904 N. Druid Hills Road #130
Decatur, GA 30033

This book is a source of information only. The author does not prescribe using any of the techniques to treat medical conditions without the advice of a physician. The author and publisher disclaim any liability for adverse effects resulting from the use or application of the information presented herein.

This book is intended for people with no complicating illness who want to lose ten to thirty pounds. Those considered obese or under medical care for any reason should work with their doctors in carrying out any weight-loss program. The information regarding home testing and remedies is for discussion purposes only. It should not be considered a replacement for medical testing, diagnosis, and treatment.

Designed by Sandra Jonas

Printed in the United States of America
18 17 16 15 14 13   1 2 3 4 5 6

Publisher's Cataloguing-in-Publication Data
Langston, Margianna.
   Unleash the thin within : the spirit, mind, and body solution to permanent weight loss / Margianna Langston — Decatur, GA : HBS Strategies Inc., 2013.
      p. : ill. ; cm.
      ISBN: 9780989057547
      Includes bibliographical references.
      1. Weight loss — Psychological aspects. 2. Mind and body.
3. Spirituality.
RM222.2 .L285 2013   613.25 — dc23
2013903725

I lovingly dedicate this book to Carolyn and Goetz, who inspire me with their unwavering courage, optimism, and cheerfulness. Thank you for your love and support of family and friends and service to God through your charitable work. You make me want to be a better person.

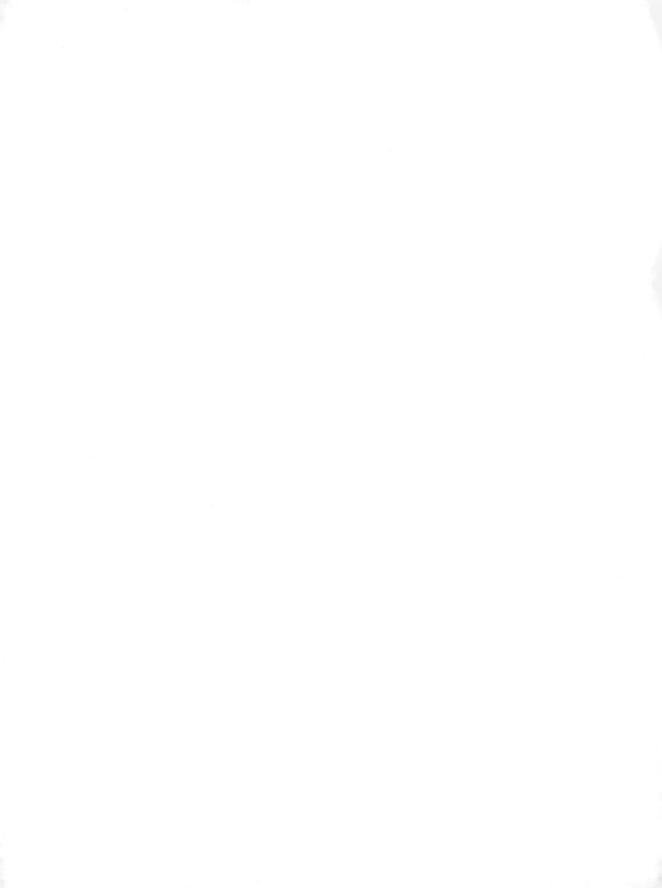

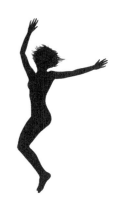

Contents

Contents

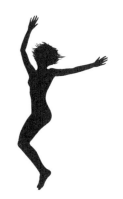

To the Reader

still recall not liking myself when I was young. In fact, I hated how I looked! I dreamed of being like my pretty, petite sister. She had an attractive, upturned nose and a flawless complexion. She also had a pleasant disposition. But it wasn't meant to be for me.

When I was eleven, I was pudgy. I had a face full of freckles and an "aristocratic" nose that looked too large to me. I was a high-strung, unhappy child with chronic headaches, sinus problems, and allergies. I frequently had a severe cough. Because of my sugar addiction, I couldn't keep my hand out of the cookie jar and, when no one was looking, stuffed slice after slice of white bread into my mouth.

College was fun, although I destroyed my body further with unhealthy habits. I burned the candle at both ends: I went out every night, smoked, ate banana splits and other sugary treats daily, and stayed up late studying for exams. One month after graduating and leaving this harmful lifestyle, I married and within the next year had a baby. By this point in my life, my body had suffered severe insult and was not functioning well, resulting in fainting spells.

In my twenties, I wandered aimlessly, searching for happiness, self-esteem, and good health. I became the president of civic clubs and the women's organization of my husband's trade association. I was active in multiple philanthropic causes and became a "somebody" for a short time.

During this frantic activity, I continued to exhaust my body, ending in a physical collapse that made it difficult for me to function. Periods of depression and feelings of hopelessness followed. The down periods were not only unpleasant but also very painful.

Now, when I look back, I realize that all my hardships were invaluable: they taught me important lessons and gave me opportunities for personal growth.

This book presents the culmination of the experiences that led to my good health and happiness. The spiritual, mental, and physical processes I developed enabled me to maintain my ideal weight and feel better about myself. This synergistic approach to weight loss incorporates universal principles that help with other self-improvement goals as well.

My prayer is that the lessons from my life will benefit you in yours. By learning how to love yourself and live a more fulfilling life, you will be on the path to your own spiritual, mental, and physical well-being. And if your goal is to lose weight, the steps I've outlined here will make it possible for you to not only shed those extra pounds but keep them off—forever.

Make no mistake: The no-diet solution in the pages ahead is not a quick fix. For me, it was only through much trial and error that I learned to incorporate the basic principles that make this wellness and happiness guide and weight management program successful.

Remember, it took many years to become the person you are today. It is essential to recognize that significant, lasting change may take time and involves creating new beliefs and behaviors to replace the outdated ones that no longer serve you. Meticu-lous practice of each step of my program will help you develop a strong, permanent foundation. This is critical if you are to avoid relapsing into old thoughts and behaviors.

One final caveat: Your result will be proportional to your commitment. Congratulations on your willingness to begin a new, exciting adventure.

With my sincere desire for your success,

Margianna

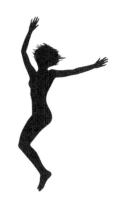

Acknowledgments

To the many people who have guided and participated with me on my life's journey, I owe my heartfelt gratitude. I would like to shine a spotlight on those who have been instrumental in my spirit, mind, and body growth:

Neil Sommerman, MD, for trusting me to develop clinical nutrition as part of his medical practice

Tony Robbins, for showing me that the impossible is possible through the fire-walk experience

Pam Watson and Robin Giles Stein, for taking me under their wings and helping me achieve success in a corporate global business

Chris Allers and Protip Biswas, for being extraordinary examples of unselfish giving in the nonprofit world and unfailingly supporting me in our work together

The staff of Sukyo Mahikari (True Light) Spiritual Development Center, for teaching me the many ways to serve God in my daily life and the value of gratitude in creating a better world.

Thank you to my friend Lynda Mattison for planting the seeds for this book by asking my thoughts on weight loss and participating in the resulting test project.

My friend Susan Hambrick will always have a special place in my heart as I remember her with love and gratitude. She helped get this book off the ground by working on the initial edit until illness intervened. It was with great sadness and sense of loss that I, her family, and other friends said a final good-bye to Susan in 2012.

Sandra Jonas, who edited, designed, and formatted *Unleash the Thin Within*, has been a godsend. She has gone beyond the call of duty to ensure the success of the book and, more importantly, to make me happy.

George Beattie, a friend and creative poet, has offered encouragement, advice, and opinions (only when asked) on the book's content and format. Thank you, George, for being my sounding board and to my other friends who inspire and cheer me on as I pursue my passions—you know who you are.

What a blessing that I have a devoted family—Earl, Rita and Jacob, Stephanie, Desiree and Nicole, Carolyn and Goetz, Smoot and Martha, Laurie and Elaine and Goetz Jr., to name a few—who love and support me no matter what, even when they disagree with my politics or think I'm weird!

Most of all, I'm grateful to God for allowing me to enjoy a wonderful, fulfilling life.

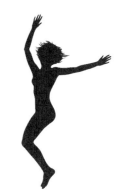

Introduction

Recall some of your diet attempts and results. Do any of these diets sound familiar?

- High-protein diet

- Complex-carbohydrate diet

- Milk-shake diet

Don't forget calorie counting and the popular prepackaged meal and fat-elimination diets.

Have you ever reached and maintained your desired weight by dieting? Do you know someone who has? Inevitably, the same theme surfaces:

I have tried every kind of diet imaginable. I lose ten pounds (or thirty), and before I can say 'plus size,' the weight returns, pound by pound, inch by inch.

Once my friends stop dieting, it is as though inner gremlins begin shouting with glee, "We can eat again! We can eat again!"

Every serial dieter knows this vicious cycle:

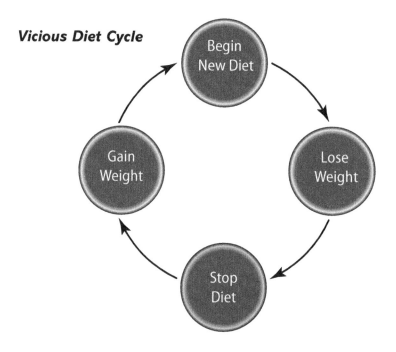

Vicious Diet Cycle

Diets Do Not Work

The truth is that weight-loss diets set you up for disappointment. When you go from one diet to the next, you live with feelings of frustration and failure on a daily basis. This ongoing disappointment leads dieters to believe that being overweight is unavoidable for them. They conclude, "I have a faulty metabolism" or "Obesity runs in my family" or "If I look at food, I gain weight." All of these may be true but aren't inevitable.

Many dieters secretly think that permanent weight loss is an impossible dream. Don't buy into this misguided logic. It is time to change your thinking and your results.

Achieve and Maintain Your Healthy Weight

Is permanent weight loss an unattainable dream? Often we judge situations in our life as impossible to change because of what we learned. Or maybe we've been burned . . .

For example, everyone knows that if you touch hot coals in a barbecue grill, you will get burned. Or will you?

Author and inspirational speaker Anthony Robbins taught me it was possible to not only touch hot coals or burning wood but also walk barefoot across them without getting burned. In the 1980s, in Atlanta and elsewhere, I completed many fire walks, including a forty-foot walk over hot mesquite wood. Although I could feel the heat, my feet didn't burn. In fact, all but one of the other two hundred participants that day successfully walked on those same coals without getting burned.

(I witnessed the paramedics tending to the badly burned feet of a man who attempted to walk over the burning wood but lost his concentration. He failed to employ the techniques Robbins taught us—ironically, this individual's misfortune proved that the coals were indeed hot and not trickery or an illusion.)

The powerful, transformative experience of walking on hot fire opened my eyes. In a matter of minutes, my mindset shifted to incorporate the belief that walking on fire was now in the realm of what was possible, rather than impossible.

Likewise, to succeed with this spirit, mind, and body approach to weight loss, it is imperative that you learn how to let go of self-limiting, negative beliefs. It is time to embrace new paradigms of what can happen.

Challenge Your Beliefs

It is up to each of us to decide if we are content with life as it is: our feelings, self-image, and appearance. If we're not okay with the status quo, then changes are in order. But our old belief systems have a habit of getting in the way.

Long-held convictions are often difficult obstacles to conquer. With regard to health, many people contend that inherited conditions are impossible to overcome or change. They'll say, "My illness is caused by my genes."

My experience is that body chemistry can be changed, regardless of family history, and that good health, along with a pleasing body, is achievable.

As I mentioned, I was a sickly, nervous child with headaches, allergies, and sugar cravings. It wasn't until I reached adulthood and enjoyed better health that I began to realize how bad I felt when growing up.

Many of these ailments occurred in my family. And so even as an adult, I believed that I was stuck with my heredity and predispositions to certain illnesses. Consequently, I took medication to control my symptoms rather than looking for the underlying causes.

Over time, I came to recognize that my belief system had led me to subconsciously make poor diet and behavioral choices. Understanding the role that spirit, mind, and body play in illness helped me adopt healthier habits. Spiritual teachings, mind exercises, professional guidance, nutritional counseling, and alternative medicine all contributed to my achieving good health. I am now well, energetic, and happy. I exhibit few signs of the debilitating allergies and addictions that I once thought were my inescapable heritage.

One day I simply decided, "I don't get sick." For over twenty-five years after that, I had no common illnesses, such as colds, flu, fever, and diarrhea.

But as I continued on my quest for spiritual, mental, and physical health, I discovered that some of what we call sickness is nature's means of purging the body of toxins and impurities to maintain health. This process is referred to as cleansings.

For instance, scientists know that a fever destroys bacteria and viruses. In fact, heating the blood to create artificial fever has been used to eliminate cancerous cells.

Although my illness-free years are proof of the mind's power, my well-intentioned commitment sometimes prevented my body

> I came to recognize that my belief system had led me to subconsciously make poor diet and behavioral choices.

from healing itself naturally. Once I became aware that my "I don't get sick" decision might be harmful, I offered a prayer to allow cleansings if they were necessary to my spiritual, mental, and physical health. The very next day—after I'd lived without sniffles for twenty-five years—my nose started running!

Warning: The mind is a powerful tool! Be thoughtful about the decisions you make so the results are consistent with your goals.

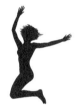

About Cleansings

A friend of mine challenged my wisdom in asking for sickness. She didn't understand why I abandoned my "I don't get sick" resolve. And she wondered why I would want so-called illness, now known as cleansings.

For decades, my body has been assaulted by over-the-counter and prescription drugs; foods containing preservatives, dyes, sugars and other chemicals; toxins in the air; stress; and negative emotions. My spirit, mind, and body suffered damage from the years I lived an unhealthy lifestyle.

If I don't allow cleansings—that is, the discharge of these toxins naturally—will this damage eventually surface as a disease, chronic illness, or life-threatening condition? I don't know. I do know that I choose to allow nature's healing mechanisms to support me in having good health. Additionally, I do my part by no longer bombarding my body with destructive influences that then require severe cleansings.

As an adult, I have never had a weight problem. I attribute my ability to maintain my weight to being extremely unhappy with myself when I was a pudgy, young teenager. At that time, I evidently decided on a subconscious level that I would never be overweight again. Since then, I have often repeated, affirmed, and, most importantly, believed that "I don't gain weight."

Thus, I have maintained my weight—even when I was diagnosed with an underactive thyroid, the leading symptom of which is weight gain.

Our Power Lies Within

My mother often lamented that it was too bad her children couldn't sing like their father. For many years, I believed her and told myself and others, "I can't sing." But I reconsidered after a choir director emphatically said to me, "If you sing for God, you can sing." Since then, I have been singing (in tune) and mastering difficult alto parts, including the chorus of Handel's *Messiah*. I am now convinced I can sing.

> When we accept negative childhood messages as fact, we let many fallacies set limits on our lives and happiness.

When we accept negative childhood messages as fact, we let many fallacies set limits on our lives and happiness. I challenged my long-held, disabling belief about my singing voice and found immense fulfillment in my choir.

You, too, can overcome ill-conceived beliefs that you accept as truths. The lessons in this book will show you how to challenge negative self-fulfilling prophecies, including your ideas about weight loss, and how to triumph over them.

Synergistic Trio

A holistic spirit, mind, and body approach is the secret to achieving the changes you desire. Think of these three as a synergistic trio intertwined like the threads of woven fabric. While each part has a separate role to play, a balanced program that focuses on the total you yields far better results.

To enjoy permanent success and peace of mind, it is important to incorporate universal spiritual principles, but I am not referring to religion or religious doctrine. Universal spiritual principles, such as gratitude, are common to most religions. The more gratitude we have for who we are and what we have, the more abundance, opportunities, and success we attract.

Most of us don't realize the power of the mind to achieve our goals—or to bring about failure. It is critical that our subconscious beliefs—what we think on a deep level—align with who we want to be, what we want to accomplish, and how we want to live our lives. To realize our dreams, we must establish this congruency.

Poor physical health can sabotage success and lead to frustrating stagnation. When we lack energy, have a fuzzy mind or persistent pain, and generally feel "bad," motivation takes a dive or disappears altogether. Needless to say, we must adopt behaviors that promote health and vibrancy. Consequently, attention to the body is another vital component of a holistic weight-loss approach.

You can lose weight and keep it off! Could it be more difficult than walking on fire?

Let's begin.

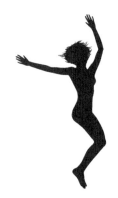

The Philosophy

Achieving weight loss is ultimately about overcoming the self-limitations that keep you in shackles and prevent the beautiful masterpiece within you from emerging.

Will you ever fully discover or complete your masterpiece? I hope not, because life is a journey. If you choose to stop, you die—if not literally, then figuratively.

Go forward with determination and commitment to become your true self.

Which Are You?

Overweight people generally fall into one of three categories:

1. **Content.** If you are twenty pounds overweight and like yourself the way you are, then you don't have a problem (unless the excess pounds create a health hazard for you). Your weight is your choice.

2. **Self-pitying.** If you see yourself as a victim of life's circumstances, then weight loss, happiness, and success will continue to elude you—unless you learn to take responsibility for yourself.

3. **Unhappy but empowered.** If you desperately want to lose weight because you have health concerns or don't feel good about yourself—or both—*and* you're willing to take charge of your life, the methods presented here will help you create permanent change.

This spirit, mind, and body approach provides the most benefits to individuals who understand that their lives are a result of their choices. They continually set goals, accept challenges, and choose to grow.

If you have the discipline to follow this entire program, you will lose weight. You can also look forward to experiencing positive life changes that may actually be more important than the weight you lose!

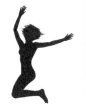

You Have a Choice

You can decide to grow up or you can hide behind the excuse that you had an unhappy childhood (or any other excuse).

You are an adult now. Your past history is just that—past history.

Each day is an opportunity to create a new history and a new life.

The Voice of God

I believe that a universal mind, known to me as God, is directing our lives. I also believe that if we pay attention, we will constantly receive guidance and messages from him.

Think about the times you have enjoyed being outside in

nature, perhaps walking in the woods on a beautiful day. How many times have you been wrestling with a problem and the solution pops into your mind without any conscious thought?

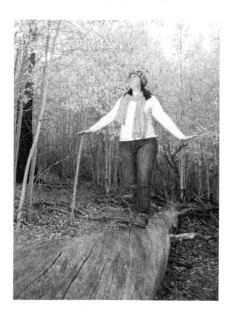

(Creative people will tell you that ideas come to them when they least expect them.)

Also, have you ever noticed that people seem to show up out of the blue when you need them most? They may tell you something profound, offer a helping hand, provide needed information, or comfort you in a time of despair.

When I was laid off during the corporate downsizing of the company I dearly loved, I was shocked and hurt. Still, as tears streamed down my face, I acknowledged to my beloved supervisor and the human resources representative that everything happens for a reason. I had no clue what the discharge meant or where it would lead but knew it was the voice of God taking me somewhere else.

(Quite truthfully, even though I recognized the voice of God throughout this painful experience, it did not lessen my anxiety about becoming unemployed. I had not yet learned to "follow the flow.")

As it turned out, the voice of God led me into the nonprofit field, a career change that gave me immeasurable satisfaction and helped facilitate the writing of this book.

I have learned that there are no accidental or lucky coincidences. Everything is the arrangement of God. Open your eyes and ears and be guided each step of the way.

Have you ever noticed that people seem to show up out of the blue when you need them most?

> ## *God's Plan*
>
>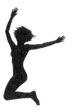
>
> You may not be able to foresee God's plan, but it is possible to develop the ability to recognize his voice. When you tune in and pay attention, you will recognize that . . .
>
> - Your intuitive thoughts guide you.
>
> - Circumstances and situations give you information and direct your path.
>
> - People appear in your life bringing you messages.
>
> By cultivating your powers of observation and intuitive skills, you will discover that help is always near. It's up to you to recognize each opportunity. Your success is waiting for you to find it.

Yes, You Can!

Don't sell yourself short. The only thing holding you back is your self-imposed limitations. Wipe the slate clean, start from zero, and accept that anything is possible.

There was a time when the brightest minds in the athletic world believed that it was impossible to run a mile in four minutes. One athlete, however, chose to ignore those naysayers, refusing to be governed by history—and he ran a four-minute mile. He proved that what most people felt was impossible was possible. After his success, other athletes changed their beliefs and ran a four-minute mile.

The current world record of 3:43.13 was set by Hicham El Guerrouj of Morocco, on July 7, 1999, in Rome.

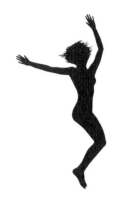

The Format

The *Unleash the Thin Within* program is divided into ten levels, each with several critical steps. To ensure your success as you move forward, practice every step precisely as written and in sequential order. It is essential that you repeat each one until it becomes a habit before progressing to the next.

The collective spirit, mind, and body develop over a lifetime. When you establish a goal to change part of the core self, your subconscious beliefs may resist your new resolve. The more ingrained those non-supportive beliefs, the greater the persistence needed to reach your goal.

The step-by-step format gives you time to accept and integrate new concepts and patterns of thought and change behaviors. This process strengthens the likelihood of permanent change and success.

For example, if a woman believes on a deep level that body metabolism slows after the age of forty, which causes weight gain, her subconscious belief becomes a self-fulfilling prophecy. People with such a mindset will struggle to lose weight and keep it off after reaching forty unless they adopt a more positive belief system.

Perhaps this could be a new belief: "My metabolism operates at optimum efficiency all my life."

Following the set of steps at each level, I present information on related topics to give you a better understanding of the recommended actions. To help you stay on course and keep track of your progress, see appendix B for review charts listing the steps for every level.

Resistance: A Deal Breaker

In this context, resistance is an internal belief that doesn't align with a specific goal. It manifests by setting up obstacles that prevent changes from taking place. In other words, resistance can sabotage your weight-loss or maintenance plan.

Understanding the three models of resistance will help you reduce it in your life:

1. No-Win Resistance

2. Win-Win Resistance

3. Quantum Leap

Identifying chaos and its role in your failure to reach goals is the first step in overcoming it.

NO-WIN RESISTANCE

Resistance or chaos in this model is a direct consequence of setting a goal that is incompatible with your internal mindset or belief. Identifying chaos and its role in your failure to reach goals is the first step in overcoming it.

Although it appears in many forms, we typically don't recognize resistance when it's occurring. Here are some signs you may encounter as you embark on this weight-loss journey:

- Suddenly being too busy to practice the weekly steps

- Becoming convinced that the program doesn't work

- Feeling depressed, confused, or negative

Other examples of chaos and resistance (forms of self-sabotage) include the following:

- Eating destructive foods

- Overeating

- Forgetting to practice the steps in this program

- Feeling sick, tired, or unmotivated

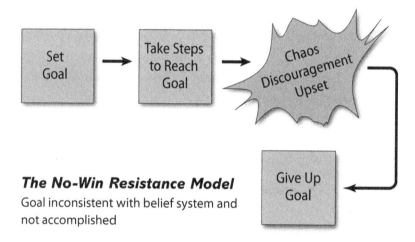

The No-Win Resistance Model
Goal inconsistent with belief system and
not accomplished

Many years ago, I wanted to start my own business, but as I took steps to realize my goal, I developed severe hypoglycemia and allergies. I experienced headaches, a foggy head, exhaustion, and depression, forcing me to put my plans on hold. With each incident, I vowed to return to my goal as soon as I was well.

Unfortunately, this cycle went on for years (manifesting itself in all areas of my life) before I finally recognized the destructive pattern. Eventually, I was able to start my business, but only after I changed my method of establishing and working toward my goals.

WIN-WIN RESISTANCE

I learned that I needed to break up my goals into small, non-threatening subgoals to avoid instances of crippling resistance. With practice, I worked to reach each subgoal, sequentially, until I reached my ultimate objective.

This is the same goal-setting methodology I advocate here. As you set and achieve mini-goals, you are taking progressive steps toward changing your beliefs and achieving your weight goal—without invoking the wrath of debilitating resistance.

The secret to doing this is to trick your mind so it won't become aware that your beliefs and life are undergoing significant changes. This is the reason for introducing changes slowly.

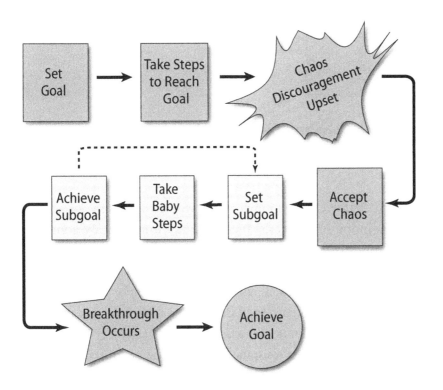

Trick your mind so it won't become aware that your beliefs and life are undergoing significant changes.

The Win-Win Resistance Model
Goal inconsistent with belief system but accomplished

The step-by-step approach in the pages ahead will help you prevail over the insidious forces of resistance. This effort will require commitment and discipline.

THE QUANTUM LEAP MODEL

Sometimes people simply establish a goal, take action to accomplish it, and immediately achieve it. In these cases, the goal is achieved in a quantum leap (almost in a single bound). This is possible when the objective is consistent with what individuals already believe is possible. Therefore, they don't experience any resistance.

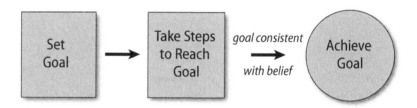

The Quantum Leap Model
Goal consistent with belief—minor or no resistance

How can you know if you will accomplish your goal with minimal or no resistance—a quantum leap? By considering your history.

In the past, if you set a weight-loss goal, dieted, and then gave up before reaching your desired weight or gained the weight back once you stopped dieting, chances are this goal is not aligned with your subconscious belief system.

To overcome resistance to your renewed effort to lose weight, be sure to patiently follow the baby steps outlined in this book and proceed gradually.

Slow Is Good and Slower Is Better!

This spirit, mind, and body approach to weight loss is designed to integrate your entire being to achieve success. As you take the journey through this book, you will create change in . . .

- Alignment with spiritual principles (spirit)

- Conscious thoughts and subconscious beliefs (mind)

- Metabolism (body)

Keep this in mind as you proceed:

- All the steps and exercises are to be practiced until you have fully integrated them into your life. Move to the next level *only* after the current level's steps become second nature.

- Use restraint and avoid peaking at future steps.

- All steps are meant to be simple and serve as part of a whole. Each step may seem insignificant when examined by itself but is synergistic when combined with the others. The whole is greater than the sum of the individual steps. Results will come as you proceed incrementally.

- To minimize the effect of resistance, remember to break your ultimate weight goal into subgoals.

Move to the next level *only* after the current level's steps become second nature.

A journey of a thousand miles begins with a single step.

—Lao-tzu

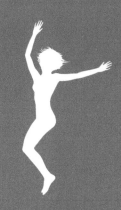

1 Believe, Pray, Commit

Working closely with a partner is absolutely essential for the program to succeed. Unless you can share your progress with someone who will support you, it will be difficult (if not impossible) to stay motivated. Remember, permanent change takes time and you will need encouragement to stick with the program and accomplish your goals.

Take Action

1.1 **Select a Partner**

Look for these characteristics in a partner:

- Positive and upbeat

- Compassionate and supportive

- Willing to always tell you the truth

- Open to giving and receiving help

- Committed to participating with you for at least six months

1

Important: Do NOT continue with this program until you find a partner.

1.2 Share Your Dreams

At the outset, you and your partner will discuss the results you want to achieve—in other words, your dreams. Focus on what you want to happen, not on what has been true in the past.

Clearly describe your desired outcome in great detail and include the following:

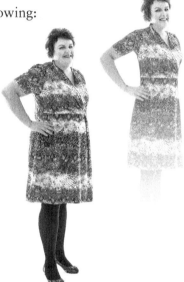

- How you will look

- How you will feel

- What it will mean to your life

Elaborate until you have nothing more to say. If you have a photograph of yourself at your desired weight, show it to your partner.

1.3 Make a Pact

You and your partner must agree to "hold each other's dreams": at all times you not only expect your partner to be successful, but imagine that his or her goals have already been reached, as in the description and picture in the previous step. It is critical to choose a partner who has no difficulty with this task because research has shown that we live up to other peoples' expectations.

1.4 Discuss Your Beliefs

Because a person's belief system is important in determining body weight, it's helpful to understand your beliefs about weight.

1

Since they're hidden in your subconscious, you can attempt to uncover them by looking for clues in your history.

Talk with your partner about your childhood and recent history and follow these guidelines:

- Were you a happy child? If not, why not?

- Are you happy now? Explain.

- When you were a child, did you overeat?

- If you are woman, was your mother—or were other female relatives—overweight?

- If you are a man, was your father—or were other male relatives—overweight?

- Did your mother or father gain weight at a particular age?

- Do you remember hearing that all women (or men) gain weight at forty years old (or at any other specific age or in a certain circumstance)?

- Do you associate good humor with being overweight person?

- How will your life change if you lose weight?

- What "bad" things do you believe will happen to you if you are more attractive?

Discuss, discuss, discuss—until you have no more to say. Don't be discouraged if your beliefs remain elusive. If you are overweight, you can assume that you need to develop new beliefs and that you will be successful following the spirit, mind, and body weight-loss program.

1

1.5 Pray for Each Other Daily

Offer a prayer every day, at a set time, for your partner. People have different concepts of prayer, so there are no specific guidelines, nor is there a suggested format. It doesn't matter how you do it, just as long as you focus on tapping into a universal power as you pray for your partner.

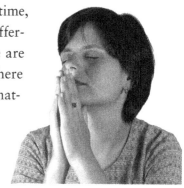

1.6 Communicate Weekly

To maintain momentum and ensure steady progress, talk (preferably meet) with your partner at least once a week. It's better to set aside the same day and time—for example, during lunch hour at work every Thursday. Use these guidelines at your meetings:

- Report the results of your practice of each step when you check in with your partner.

- Perform the exercises that involve your partner, allowing time before or after the meeting to socialize.

- Congratulate each other on your successes.

- Decide if you are ready to advance to the next level (and do so only if both of you are consistently practicing all the steps in the previous level).

- In addition to planned meetings, call your partner whenever you need help or encouragement.

1.7 Cheer Each Other On

- Empower and encourage your partner to continue.

- Have the attitude of "You can do it!"

1

- Refrain from beating yourself up (and don't allow your partner to beat herself up) if you haven't carried out the steps perfectly.

- Focus on your accomplishments.

1.8 **Commit to Your Goals**

Memorize William H. Murray's commitment passage (page 31) before your next weekly meeting.

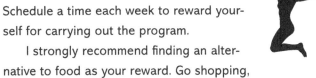

Reward

Schedule a time each week to reward your-self for carrying out the program.

I strongly recommend finding an alter-native to food as your reward. Go shopping, take in a movie or relax reading a novel.

If your reward absolutely has to be a decadent food, so be it. Just remember the consequences and decide if you're willing to suffer them.

Research and Discussion

Hazel was thirty-eight years old and fifty pounds overweight. I asked her to tell me about her life.

"I've been married for thirteen years," she said. "I have a good job and I'm very active in our church." Except for being overweight, she was happy. She wanted to lose weight, but she'd had no success with past dieting attempts.

During our conversation, I asked her if she had ever been

1

slim. She said that as a teenager, she was very attractive and had a normal weight. When I asked her to describe her life at that time, she said that needing attention from men consumed her. She equated this attention with being loved, and she slept around a lot.

Her promiscuity led to having a baby out of wedlock. Those were difficult years, Hazel told me, because she had to drop out of school to support herself and her child.

The more we talked, the more Hazel became aware of her internal belief system. She finally said that she associated being slim and attractive with being sinful.

It is no wonder that Hazel had trouble losing weight. Her deep faith made it unacceptable to be the person she was as a teenager. Her fear of going against her religious beliefs was controlling her appearance and keeping her overweight.

Hazel needed to replace the negativity she attributed to being attractive with a more positive mindset. I asked her, "What are some of the benefits to losing weight? Think in terms of your spiritual, mental, and physical well-being and your ability to help others."

After giving this question a lot of thought, Hazel said, "My health would improve, I would live longer and have more energy to work for our church, and my husband would find me more attractive."

I asked her to make a list of the benefits and continue adding to it as she thought of more. I also gave her exercises to help the process of changing her internal beliefs and assured her that she would eventually be able to reach her goal weight.

Belief as a Mental Force

A group of graduate students at a major university was assigned the task of helping students at a local middle school achieve better grades.

1

The investigators announced that they were placing the "best" students from the three fifth-grade classes in a class together. Then they assigned the "best" teacher to this class. At the beginning of the school year, all students in the three fifth-grade classes were given standardized tests.

During the school year, the best students in their separate class and the average students in the other two classes were taught from the same curriculum and the same books. At the end of the school year, all three classes were tested again. As expected by parents and educators, the "best" class with the "best" teacher excelled, far outscoring the students in the other classes.

Then the graduate students revealed all the details of their experiment. The teachers, parents, and students were shocked to learn that the average scores of all three classes on the original tests were virtually identical, and that the "best" students and the "best" teacher were actually selected through a random drawing of all fifth-grade students and teachers!

These results clearly demonstrate how expectations play a big part in our success. The students and teacher chosen as the "best" believed they were the best. So with this belief and accompanying expectations, the students learned quickly and easily.

Schools that establish high expectations for all students—and provide the support necessary to meet those expectations—have high rates of academic success.

If you believe you are unattractive or unlovable, your perception will be your reality. If you expect to gain positive results from this program, you will. I believe that you are the best student, that I am the best teacher of this subject matter, and that you are attractive and lovable. You *will* be able to change your mind and your life.

With my guidance, you'll become convinced that you are lovable and attractive. I will hold the dream knowing that you possess these qualities and that someday you will believe it is true.

If you expect to gain positive results from this program, you will.

1

The power of prayer in healing (along with the role of a higher being) has long been questioned by science.

The Power of Prayer

Traditionally, prayer has not been a component of mainstream medicine or science. Despite witnessing miracle cures and healings, many doctors have done their best to use other reasons to explain these experiences. The power of prayer in healing (along with the role of a higher being) has long been questioned by science, because scientific thinking requires unequivocal, physical proof.

Beginning in 1982, double-blind studies were performed to prove or disprove the benefit of prayer in healing. Cardiologist Larry Dossey is one of the doctors and researchers who led the way in this research. He assembled 393 heart patients and randomly divided them into two groups. From August 1982 until May 1983, one group was the subject of organized prayer and the other group was not. The study did not ask family members and friends not to pray for those in the "no prayer" group.

No one connected to the patients (that is, the doctors, nurses, other hospital staff, patients, patients' families, and the study director) knew how the patients had been divided up. People belonging to prayer groups were sent notices asking them to pray for a particular patient. Both groups of patients received identical medical care.

At the end of the ten-month study, members of the experimental group were healthier than those in the control group. Patients who had received prayers had exhibited less need for CPR, mechanical ventilators, diuretics, and antibiotics, and experienced lower rates of pulmonary edema and fewer deaths.

Dossey's study results could not be explained scientifically. Nevertheless, the only variable was prayer.

Skeptics may claim that studies showing the efficacy of prayer are somehow skewed by human input, bias, or the placebo effect, but research performed on nonhuman living organisms has yielded similar results.

1

Europeans have examined the power of prayer on enzyme cells, bacteria, plants, and animals. In one study, prayer groups were assigned to pray for plant growth. At points throughout the same study, the groups were directed to pray *against* plant growth. The findings revealed that plant growth responded according to the focus of the prayers.

In another study, Dr. Franklin Loehr, a scientist and Presbyterian minister, measured the effects of prayer on germinating seeds. In one experiment, he grew three pans of various kinds of seeds: a control pan, a "positive prayer" pan, and a "negative prayer" pan.

The results indicated that the positive-prayer seeds germinated more quickly and produced more vigorously than the plants growing in the other pans. Among the negative-prayer plants, some experienced halted germination and others suppressed growth. While plants in the control pan grew, they grew more slowly than those receiving positive prayers.

Other experiments on seeds and plants have yielded similar findings.

In his book *Love Thyself: The Message from Water III*, Dr. Masaru Emoto provides tangible evidence of the influence that our thoughts, words, and prayers have on our world. He explains:

> *How can we know how the power of prayer works? I can't explain the mechanism. The one thing I can say with confidence is that when it works in the water, it can actually alter its structure.*
>
> *This means that we've proven that physical energy can change in accordance with our wishes. I've become absolutely convinced of this after carrying out so many experiments where we've prayed over water and actually transformed its crystals into more beautiful forms.*

The findings revealed that plant growth responded according to the focus of the prayers.

Below are two examples from Dr. Emoto's research. Photographs were taken before and after a group of people prayed over samples of water from the heavily polluted Lake Carapicuiba near Sao Paulo, Brazil. After the water was frozen, Dr. Emoto viewed the resulting crystalline structures under a microscope. This is what he saw:

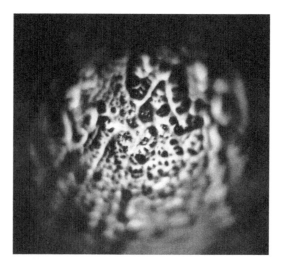

Water crystal before prayer at Lake Carapicuiba

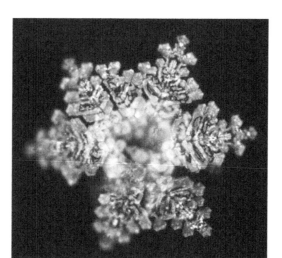

Water crystal after prayer at Lake Carapicuiba

1

Pray with Your Feet Running

I have often heard the story about a man who prayed to God to win the lottery. For many months, he offered this prayer to win the lottery but nothing happened. Fed up with God's lack of response, he berated him, "I've prayed over and over again for this one thing, but you have ignored me. I really don't know if you answer prayers or even exist."

Finally, he heard a voice clearly say, "My dear child, I love you and want to give you everything that will make you happy. However, you've got to do your part. You've asked to win the lottery over and over again, and you are angry with me because it has not happened. If you want to win the lottery, you must first buy a ticket."

I cannot change you, nor can anyone else. You must change yourself by taking the steps that will get you to your goals.

Commitment Is a Prerequisite

Many years ago, I was one of 250 participants at Marshall Thurber's Future of Business seminar in Colorado. We were divided into small groups and given William H. Murray's passage about commitment to learn and recite to the entire assembly.

I was extremely embarrassed because I couldn't memorize the short passage, despite having been an honor student in school. My compassionate teammates decided we should present it in unison as a show of support for me.

1

After the event, I reflected on why I couldn't learn the material. I realized that I didn't want to commit to any direction in my life because I was afraid of making mistakes. The fact that I was recently divorced and my life was in disarray played a huge part in my subconscious decision to make no commitments. "Footloose and fancy-free" was my motto.

But in time I began setting and reaching new goals, and my life smoothed out. At that point, I learned the commitment passage with ease.

Several years later, when I was a guest teacher in the summer-long Governor's Honor Program in Georgia, I taught goal setting and achievement principles. A limited number of academically superior high school students who also demonstrated extraordinary leadership skills were chosen to participate. For a homework assignment, I gave them Murray's commitment piece to memorize.

The following day, I asked the group of students sitting together at each table to recite the passage with their tablemates. The groups did so, flawlessly, with the exception of two students. These engaging young men said that they were not sure they remembered all of it. So I instructed them to stand on top of the table and say the passage together, and the class would help if needed.

This exercise turned out to be incredibly memorable. The boys stood on the table, looked at each other, and proceeded to recite everything perfectly, adding an impromptu dramatization of each sentence. They were priceless and fearless. They knew the material but lacked confidence.

The students in the Governor's Honors Program understood commitment—perhaps that is why they excelled in school. I imagine that your ability or willingness to memorize the passage is an indication of the ease or difficulty you have in committing to weight loss.

1

Commitment

"Until one is committed, there is hesitancy, the chance to draw back, always ineffectiveness.

Concerning all acts of initiative (and creation), there is one elementary truth, the ignorance of which kills countless ideas and splendid plans: that the moment one definitely commits oneself, then Providence moves too.

All sorts of things occur to help one that would otherwise never have occurred. A whole stream of events issues from the decision, raising in one's favor all manner of unforeseen incidents, meetings and material assistance, which no man could have dreamt would have come his way.

I learned a deep respect for one of Goethe's couplets:

Whatever you can do or dream you can, begin it.
Boldness has genius, power and magic in it!"

—William H. Murray, *The Scottish Himalayan Expedition*

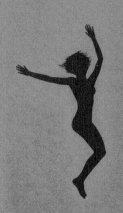

A Better Way to Eat 2

Evaluate your commitment to success and the benefits you want to achieve. Then ramp up your metabolism to aid your body in burning calories, replacing fat with muscle, and increasing your energy by incorporating the following habits and food into your daily routine.

Take Action

2.1 **Review Level 1**

2.2 **Discuss the Commitment Passage**
Talk about the meaning of the passage and your ease or difficulty in memorizing it.

2.3 **Encourage Successful Outcomes**
Brainstorm and write down the positive benefits of losing weight and then prioritize the items on your list to determine the top three. Without fail, write down the top three benefits in longhand each night immediately before going to sleep.

Continue adding to your list and reprioritizing as you think of additional benefits.

Margianna Langston

2.4 **Increase Your Metabolism with New Eating Habits**

- **Eat often and in small quantities.** "Small" is the key word. When you eat six meals a day, your total food intake should not exceed the amount you would eat in two or three meals a day. As you make this new meal pattern a part of your daily life, you will be amazed by how much more energy you will have and, as your hunger decreases, how much weight you will lose. See below for suggested foods to include in your six meals.

- **Consume quality foods.** Select items from this list to include in your mini-meals:

  - Nuts and seeds: almonds, macadamias, walnuts, pistachios, and sunflower seeds

  - Hummus, guacamole, or salsa on rice crackers

  - Yogurt and kefir (no or low sugar)

  - Natural cheese, including cottage cheese

  - Hard-boiled eggs

  - Fruit: apples, pears, mangos, papaya, grapes, blueberries, and figs

  - Leafy greens: leaf lettuce, bok choy, parsley, cilantro, spinach, kale, and spring greens

  - Other vegetables: raw or steamed broccoli florets, carrots, kale, celery, cauliflower, cucumbers, miniature red and yellow peppers, and onions

  - Chicken or beef

  - Edame (soybeans)

2

- ☐ Salmon, tuna, sardines, and other wild fish—baked or patties

- ☐ Beans: soups or dishes with lentils, black beans and/or quinoa with beneficial spices (garlic, onions, turmeric, cumin, cayenne pepper)

- ☐ Uncrystallized ginger pieces soaked and rinsed to remove sugar

- ☐ Protein drinks

- **Time your meals.** Consume the majority of your calories early in the day. Decrease your caloric intake as the day progresses. Try to eat little, or preferably nothing at all, after your evening meal.

- **Avoid refined carbohydrates.** Your body converts carbohydrates into glucose, which is then converted to fuel, making carbs essential to normal functioning. However, when you consume excess quantities, the body stores them as fat and causes you to crave more sugar, leading to the tendency to overeat.

  Limit carbs to those found naturally in foods (fruit, for example) and avoid refined forms, such as desserts, candies, sodas, breads, pasta, rice, and juices. Particularly harmful are foods that contain sucrose and high fructose corn syrup. Such artificial sweeteners as aspartame, saccharin, and sucralose may aid in weight loss, but some experts say that these chemicals cause other health problems. The safest dietary path is to use "novel" sweeteners, such as stevia, which have no calories, or small amounts of natural sweeteners, such as honey, molasses, or maple syrup.

- **Limit saturated and trans fats.** For many years, the prevalent opinion among health professionals has been that we should

2

limit our intake of saturated fats, those fats that are solid at room temperature. Sources include animal protein, poultry, whole-fat dairy products, and margarine or other trans fats, saturated fats created when hydrogen is added to a liquid fat. According to these experts, saturated fats are stored in the body and therefore contribute to weight gain, along with such conditions as elevated cholesterol, heart disease, and stroke.

More recently, some in the medical community have expressed opposition to this conventional wisdom, contending that saturated fat does not cause obesity or other health conditions. Everyone agrees, however, that trans fats, often identified on labels as "partially hydrogenated oil," are harmful and should be eliminated from the diet.

Research and Discussion

Mini-Meals and Blood Sugar

After large meals, the spike in glucose (blood sugar) causes a large release of insulin from the pancreas, triggering the body to use some of the glucose for fuel while storing the excess amounts as fat.

In contrast, frequently eating small amounts of food maintains a low level of glucose, encouraging the body to convert all the fat into fuel. The upside to the fuel staying at a consistent level is decreased appetite and less weight gain.

Diets that severely limit calories cause the body to go into survival mode, slowing cell metabolism to preserve enough fuel to function. So when normal eating is resumed, weight gain is inevitable and becomes a chronic problem.

Mini-meals, on the other hand, will give you constant nutrients and calories to maintain an efficiently operating metabolism. Eating frequently will rev up your body and lead to weight loss.

Eating frequently will rev up your body and lead to weight loss.

It is a good idea to snack on small amounts of healthy foods all day long while eating most of your food by early afternoon. I typically eat a moderate breakfast and lunch and a smaller dinner with mini-meals or healthy snacks in between. I do not gain weight, because I consume nutritious foods in proper amounts, in the most beneficial way and, just as important, because I believe "I don't gain weight."

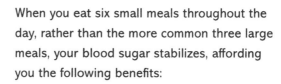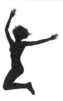

"Mini Size Me"

When you eat six small meals throughout the day, rather than the more common three large meals, your blood sugar stabilizes, affording you the following benefits:

- Reduced hunger and cravings for sweets

- Increased energy

- Weight loss

The Fats Controversy

A lot of contradictory information exists about the effects of saturated fats on our health. In a 2010 study, the Harvard School of Public Health found that replacing saturated fats with polyunsaturated fats reduced the coronary heart disease risk by 19 percent. At the same time, the American Journal of Clinical Nutrition discovered no connection between saturated fat consumption and increased risk of coronary heart disease.

Other studies and experts agree with the American Journal's conclusion. In his book *Good Calories, Bad Calories*, science writer Gary Taubes states that dietary fat does not lead to obe-

2

sity or other medical problems. Holistic practitioner Dr. Andrew Weil concurs, maintaining that the culprit is a high-carbohydrate diet, not saturated fat. Dr. Weil does believe in limiting saturated fat, though, because it replaces vitamins, minerals, and other nutrients needed for good health.

Some health professionals argue that natural-occurring, plant-based saturated fats, such as coconut oil, actually benefit the body.

But there is no disagreement about the harm caused by trans fats. They raise LDL (bad) cholesterol and lower HDL (good) cholesterol. Found in a host of processed foods, trans fats generally taste good, but they travel through the digestive system and clog the arteries.

To function properly, the body requires some dietary fat, but it's in our best interest to consume mostly unsaturated fats, such as those found in fatty fish, olive oil, nuts, seeds, and avocados, and stay away from trans fats.

Foods to Avoid

The following are five examples of the worst foods you can eat, because they lack nutritional value and contain many toxins:

1. **Doughnuts.** A store-bought doughnut is made of about 35 to 40 percent trans fat that is damaging to cells, has 200–300 calories, and can damage your blood-sugar balance. It is fried and loaded with refined sugar and white flour.

2. **Soda.** The average can of soda contains about ten teaspoons of sugar, 150 calories, from 30 mg to 55 mg of caffeine, artificial food colors, and sulfites. Studies have linked soda to osteoporosis, obesity, tooth decay, and heart disease. The average American drinks an estimated fifty-six gallons of soft drinks each year. Over the last decade, children have doubled their consumption.

Studies have linked soda to osteoporosis, obesity, tooth decay, and heart disease.

2

3. **French fries.** Anything fried in trans fat at high temperatures is dangerous because the potent cancer-causing substance acrylamide is created during the process.

4. **Chips.** Traditional corn, potato, and tortilla chips are high in trans fat. Additionally, the high-temperature cooking methods can cause the formation of carcinogenic substances, such as acrylamide.

5. **Fried seafood.** Toxic levels of mercury have been found in seafood. Shellfish, including shrimp and lobster, can be contaminated with parasites and resistant viruses (that may not be killed even with high heat). Eating fried seafood potentially exposes you to a quadruple dose of toxins: trans fat, acrylamide, mercury, and parasites or viruses. Fish caught in the wild, such as wild red Alaskan salmon, is free of many harmful contaminants. Always prepare fish using baking or grilling methods rather than frying.

(Adapted from "The Five Absolute Worst Foods You Can Eat," Dr. Joseph Mercola's natural health newsletter)

3 Gratitude Is Key

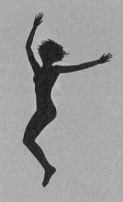

Living in a world made up of vibrations, we are creating our destiny every moment. When we experience and express gratitude, we surround ourselves with positive vibrations that have the power to change our internal chemistry.

Gratitude is an essential spiritual teaching because its presence in our thoughts, words, and actions affects the mind and body. You can use gratitude to grow spiritually and improve your life, as well as the lives of your family and friends.

A grateful mindset will open the door to success, whereas negative feelings will close it. The following neuro-linguistic programming (NLP) techniques can help you eliminate negative beliefs and learn how to live in gratitude.

> You can use gratitude to grow spiritually and improve your life, as well as the lives of your family and friends.

Take Action

3.1 **Review Level 2**

3.2 **Practice Gratitude**
When you wake up in the morning, express gratitude for such things as . . .

3

- Being alive

- A restful night's sleep

- Your family

- Your home

- Your job

- Everything and everyone else in your life

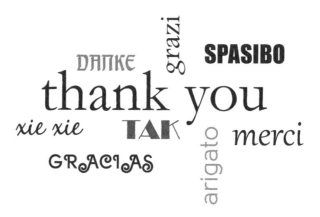

Continue expressing gratitude throughout the day (silently or aloud). Here are some examples:

- Thank you for allowing my family and me to have good health.

- Thank you for the peace and freedom I enjoy.

- Thank you for my beautiful home and my safe, reliable car.

Think of reasons to thank your coworkers. Here is one suggestion: I am grateful for all your hard work in helping me finish my project.

Express gratitude even if you don't feel grateful. Focus on what you have rather than on what you don't have. Eventually, you will recognize that you have many things to be grateful for and you will learn to live in gratitude. Gratitude is a key to happiness.

3.3 Adopt an Attitude of Gratitude for Water

Practice being grateful for everything you ingest, because the food we eat and the water we drink keep us healthy and alive.

It's especially important to focus on water:

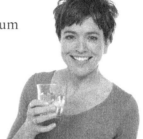

- Drink with gratitude a minimum of four ounces of water every hour.

- Keep a glass of water or a water bottle within easy reach at all times.

Read the following statements to determine which one looks, sounds, or feels best to you:

- "As I drink this water with gratitude, I visualize it flowing into every cell of my body—*nourishing, energizing, and flushing out fat*." In your mind, can you see this happening?

- "As I drink this water with gratitude, I hear the swooshing sound as it flows into every cell of my body—*nourishing, energizing, and flushing out fat*." Can you internally hear the sounds?

- "As I drink this water with gratitude, I feel it flowing into every cell of my body—*nourishing, energiz-*

3

ing, and flushing out fat." Do you feel the internal sensations?

Which statement resonates most with you? When you drink water, repeat it as you practice what it says; that is, visualize the action, hear the sound, or feel the water.

The goal of this practice is to link gratitude with the healthy habit of drinking water until your gratitude becomes automatic and your mind is reprogrammed to aid in weight loss as you drink water. Visualizing, hearing, or feeling yourself flushing out fat when you drink water will begin to influence your mind and subconscious beliefs in ways that you may not yet understand or trust.

3.4 Conquer Depression

Stop what you are doing now and feel depressed. Do this by thinking of a time in your life when you were depressed because of negative circumstances. Feel the feelings, hear what people were saying or what you were saying to yourself, and visualize the scenario.

Now, as you are experiencing the negative feelings of depression, feel and express gratitude for your life, your family, and your friends.

Is the depression still controlling you? If you are truly being grateful, you'll find it impossible to be grateful and depressed at the same time.

3.5 Determine Your Primary Learning Style

The statement you chose in 3.3 that best resonates with you can give you a clue about the primary way you perceive the world, whether it's visual, auditory, or kinesthetic. To get a more accurate idea of your style, work through the following exercises with your partner:

3

Part 1. Ask your partner each of the following questions and record how his or her eyes move during the reply:

- If a friend called you after midnight to go out to eat, what would you wear?

  Eyes _____.

- Have you ever gone out with a friend to eat after midnight?

  Eyes _____.

- How would you feel if you received a phone call after midnight from a friend asking you to go out to eat?

  Eyes _____.

Which of the eye movements below best describes your partner's eye movements?

- Up and to the right

  VISUAL
- Up and to the left

- Level and to the right

  AUDITORY
- Level and to the left

- Down and to the left   KINESTHETIC

Part 2. Check all the following characteristics that apply to you and ask your partner for his or her opinion:

3

Visual (Seeing)

- ❏ Stands tall with shoulders and head up

- ❏ Stands close and leans forward when talking

- ❏ Speaks at a fast pace with animation/gestures

- ❏ Converses clearly and colorfully, using words such as "see," "look," and "imagine"

- ❏ Likes to look attractive and pays attention to detail

- ❏ Breathes rapidly and high in the chest

- ❏ Loves order and beauty

- ❏ Moves eyes up and to the right when constructing a mental picture or trying to imagine something, and up and to the left when remembering

Auditory (Hearing)

- ❏ Loves to talk and uses words like "hear," "sound," "noise," and phrases like "rings a bell"

- ❏ Breathes in middle of chest

- ❏ Stands relaxed but with good posture

- ❏ Moves eyes laterally to the right when creating, to the left when remembering, and down and left when having internal dialogue

- ❏ Has a soothing voice

- ❏ Talks to self with internal dialogue

- ❏ Struggles with making decisions because the internal voices endlessly debate

- ❏ Often does not trust feelings

Kinesthetic (Feelings)

- ❏ Talks slowly with pauses while determining feelings about what is being said

- ❏ Uses words such as "feel," "touch," "sense," "grasp," "like," "hate," "warm," "cold," and "lukewarm"

- ❏ Breathes deeply from the belly

- ❏ Stands slumped over with the chest inward

- ❏ Moves eyes down to the left when speaking to get into feelings or bodily sensations

- ❏ Relies on intuitive feelings to make decisions

- ❏ Is sensitive to the thoughts, vibrations, and energy of others

Determine your primary thinking, learning, and communicating mode by counting up the number of checks you have under each of the categories. Keep in mind that your style is likely not limited to that one exclusively. In fact, you may change it to fit different people and situations.

As you put this awareness into practice, use the words that match your partner's style:

- • If you are visual, your partner might say to you, "I *see* that you have learned the commitment passage."

- • If you are auditory, your partner might say, "It *sounds* like you have learned the commitment passage."

- • If you are primarily kinesthetic, your partner might say, "I *feel* that it was easy for you to learn the commitment passage."

3

Using words that match the way your partner thinks, learns, and communicates will build rapport and help you better understand the instructions. To be effective, remember to address others in *their* primary mode, rather than in your own.

Research and Discussion

As mentioned, Dr. Masaru Emoto discovered that our thoughts have the power to change the world around us. The movie *What the Bleep Do We Know!?* offers more examples of his dramatic water research.

Photographs were taken of two sets of frozen water crystals: the first from clear water springs exposed to loving words and the second from water exposed to negative thoughts or pollution.

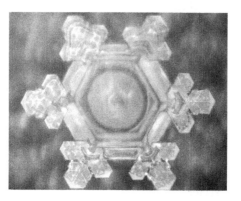

Water crystals exposed to gratitude

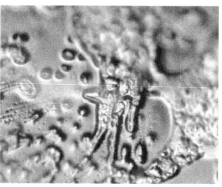

Water crystals exposed to negativity

The crystals from the water exposed to loving words were brilliant, complex, and colorful in snowflake patterns. On the other hand, crystals from polluted water and water exposed to negative thoughts were dull, incomplete, and asymmetrical.

Could this be proof that water within the cells in our body is also affected by our thoughts, feelings, and words?

While you drink water, thank the water with heartfelt appreciation for providing life to you. I believe that Emoto's research strengthens the argument for developing a constant state of gratitude.

Like Vibrations Attract

The vibrations we and others emit, positive or negative, attract similar vibrations to us, and to the greater world around us. Since like attracts like, when we express gratitude, we attract more positive forces into our lives for which to be grateful. So we have the power to create our destiny in every moment. Consider this:

- Do some people make you feel happy and empowered?

- Do other people cause your good mood to go down the tube by just being in their company?

Have you ever felt worried, unhappy, or depressed when you were experiencing gratitude? Chances are that you haven't. It's close to impossible to have negative emotions and vibrations at the same time as gratitude.

I can't say it often enough: practicing gratitude can change your moods and your life.

Reframing "Mistakes"

Adopting an attitude of gratitude means that you will never fail in the *Unleash the Thin Within* program, even if you are unable

When we express gratitude, we attract more positive forces into our lives for which to be grateful.

3

to carry out every step precisely as written. Berating yourself is not permissible. It will undermine your results.

Adopt the attitude that mistakes are learning experiences leading you to success.

Has it occurred to you to be thankful when you eat half a chocolate cake? Or do you feel guilty? Try expressing gratitude for the chocolate cake—see, hear, and feel it nourish your cells. If you do this with sincerity, the result of such an indiscretion will ultimately be positive.

Reframe your mistakes and choose to behave differently in the future.

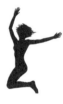

Weight Loss Tip

Think in terms of being on your way to a more fulfilling life. Share the fact that you are participating in this program only with those who will fully encourage and support you.

Appreciation for Water

The adult body is composed of approximately 60 percent water. While most people understand the importance of water, many don't understand the necessity of hydrating the body for health, including weight loss. Incredible as it may seem, water is quite possibly the single most important catalyst in losing weight and keeping it off.

Water suppresses the appetite naturally and helps the body metabolize stored fat. Studies have shown that a decrease in water intake will cause fat deposits to increase, whereas an increase in water intake can actually reduce fat deposits. When the kidneys don't have adequate water to function properly, the

3

liver must step in to help, limiting its ability to focus on converting stored fat into usable energy, the liver's primary function.

Obesity also decreases the percentage of water in the body, sometimes to as low as 45 percent. So it is even more imperative that an overweight person drink plenty of water.

Water flushes out toxins, carries nutrients to the cells, normalizes body temperature, maintains acid-alkaline balance, and helps burn calories. Even a mild case of dehydration can threaten normal body function. Some medical professionals have estimated that 75 percent of Americans are chronically dehydrated. Dehydration can cause metabolism to slow as much as 3 percent.

Thirst can be a poor way of monitoring your water needs. You can lose your thirst sensation and the critical perception of needing water. No longer recognizing a need for water, you can become gradually, increasingly, and chronically dehydrated with age. A "dry mouth" may be a late sign of dehydration.

The functions of water:

- Transports vitamins, minerals, amino acids, glucose, hormones, enzymes, digestive juices, and other substances throughout your body

- Assists chemical reactions, such as the burning of glucose and the breakdown of fat for energy

- Lubricates joints, eyeballs, nasal passages, and the intestines

- Absorbs shock for your eyes and spinal cord

- Maintains your body temperature: cools the body by evaporation from the skin and lungs and helps retain warmth in winter

- Removes wastes through the kidneys and helps solid waste pass through the intestines

Water suppresses the appetite naturally and helps the body metabolize stored fat.

3

Possible symptoms of chronic dehydration:

- Fatigue, muscle cramps, and dizziness
- Fuzzy short-term memory and difficulty focusing (can be triggered by a 2 percent decrease in hydration)
- Constipation
- Fluid retention
- Increased risk of urinary tract infections and kidney stones
- High and low blood pressure
- Excess weight and obesity
- Premature aging—shriveled and dry skin that lacks elasticity and doesn't bounce back when pinched
- Digestive disorders
- Respiratory problems
- Acid-alkaline imbalance

Conditions exacerbated by chronic dehydration:

- Heartburn and ulcers
- Diabetes
- Depression
- Allergies and asthma
- Rheumatoid arthritis
- Back pain
- Heart pain

3

- Headaches

- High blood pressure

- High cholesterol

- Leg pains

Drink More Water

- Drinking eight to ten glasses of water daily can ease back and joint pain for up to 80 percent of sufferers.

- Drinking five glasses of water daily decreases the risk of certain cancers.

- Water can shut down midnight hunger (thirst is often mistaken for hunger).

NLP: A Powerful Tool

What if changing your belief system about weight loss and maintenance became easier?

Neuro-linguistic programming (NLP) is a behavioral technology: a set of guiding principles, attitudes, and techniques about real-life behavior. While it is not science, individuals who learn to practice NLP techniques can more quickly change, adopt, or eliminate specific behaviors.

Most people have a primary mode or style that controls how they think, learn, and communicate. NLP divides these styles into five categories, or representational systems that are simply the five senses.

3

While taste and smell are important, neither is generally as dominant in controlling communication to the brain as the visual, auditory, and kinesthetic senses. Here is a brief description of how each type operates in the world:

- Visual people often respond quickly—their motto could be "ready, fire, aim."

- Auditory people analyze the pros and cons extensively before making a decision.

- Kinesthetic or feeling-dominated people make decisions from their gut.

Now that have discovered your preferred learning style, you can use that knowledge to more quickly absorb information and replace non-supportive subconscious programming with supportive programming.

Choosing to Take Control

Frankly, tapping into your subconscious and making life changes is no easy task. But it can be done.

To systematically reprogram deep-seated beliefs and change your self-image or identity, the mind must be inundated with new input. One way of doing this is to repeat an affirmation. The affirmation will be more effective if you use your visual, hearing, and feeling senses in vividly creating the stated action, such as:

- When I drink green tea, my metabolism speeds up.

- I am that slim, beautiful person in the picture.

- Fat drops off my hips with each step I take.

Each of these statements is true. For example, green tea does

3

energize the metabolism, so to enhance the affirmation, visualize yourself full of energy, hearing family and friends congratulating you and feeling a sense of satisfaction that this is something you have accomplished.

By frequently affirming that these and other statements are true, you can incorporate the power of your mind and senses to help you reach your goal. Commitment and persistence are the ingredients that make things happen.

Mind Power

Many years ago, I read about an experiment conducted by Australian psychologist Alan Richardson, who wanted to study the effects of visualization on athletic performance. He randomly selected three groups of basketball players and tested their ability to shoot a series of free throws.

For the next twenty days, the first group practiced twenty minutes a day, the second didn't practice at all, and the third group visualized shooting perfect baskets.

When Richardson tested them again, he discovered that the first group improved 24 percent, the second showed no improvement, and the third improved 23 percent, almost as much as the group that practiced. He concluded that the nervous system and mind couldn't tell the difference between an actual experience and a vividly imagined one.

Practice creating in your mind how you will look at your ideal weight.

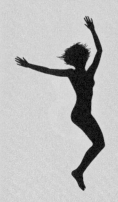

Make Over
Your Body and Mind 4

Your vision of the body, happiness, and life that you want is now becoming a reality. Your success will be assured by changing your diet, eliminating negative subconscious programming, creating a beautiful vision of yourself, and having a positive outlook. The steps in this level are an easy but essential part of your weight-loss journey.

Take Action

4.1   **Review Level 3**

4.2   **Add Essential Fatty Acids (EFAs) to Your Diet**
Eating foods containing good fat several times a week will help you lose weight, lower your risk for heart attack, and support your brain. Here are rich sources of essential fatty acids:

- Flaxseeds

- Walnuts and macadamia nuts

- Salmon

- Sardines

- Herring

- Avocados

- Eggs

- Olive oil (unheated, or heated at a low temperature)

- Flaxseed oil (do not heat)

You will notice that several of these foods are listed in the mini-meal suggestions in level 2 (page 33). Include baked or broiled salmon dishes in at least two of the meals you eat every week and try adding sardines to a tossed salad or having them alone with mustard.

Mindful Eating

- Set aside ample time for every meal.

- Use small plates and utensils.

- Express gratitude.

- Eat small bites.

- Slow down and enjoy the experience.

4.3 **Savor Everything You Eat**

The hypothalamus gland controls the hunger mechanism (appestat) in our body. It generally takes about twenty minutes to register that you have eaten enough to satisfy your hunger.

Many people overeat before they start feeling full. So slow

4

down and enjoy each small bite. Allow your appestat to catch up with your food intake.

4.4 **Change Your Image**

Find a picture of yourself at your desired weight. If you have never been your desired weight, find a full-body picture of someone in a magazine or a picture of a friend or family member at an attractive weight. Paste a headshot of yourself onto this desired body. Be realistic! Now do the following:

- Make a copy of the picture.

- Post one of the pictures in a prominent place.

- While viewing that picture, imagine stepping into it and remember how you looked and felt, what you were thinking or saying to yourself, and what other people were saying as they admired you at your desired weight. Feel the satisfaction and warmth that spreads throughout your body as you recall this memory.

- Cut the second copy of the photograph into several pieces (similar to puzzle pieces):

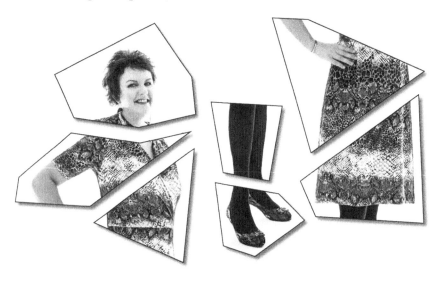

4

Tape each piece on a different item: your mirror, computer, TV, car dashboard, checkbook, weekly planner, refrigerator, billfold (anywhere you will see the pieces often).

When you see a puzzle piece, your mind will remember the entire picture and your subconscious mind over time will be inundated with this new image. Before long, you will not consciously notice the puzzle pieces, yet your subconscious will see them and they will continue to work for you.

Before falling asleep, study and admire the intact picture for five minutes while remembering all the sensations and thoughts you have associated with the picture. The picture, along with your thoughts and feelings, will sink into your subconscious while your mind is in this relaxed state. With daily practice, your subconscious mind will accept that this picture is you, and your body will begin to adjust to match this image. (See appendix C for information on accessing Virtual Weight Loss Mirror, an online tool that will create a picture of how you will look after you lose weight.)

4.5 **Pat Yourself on the Back**

When "bad" things are happening to us, it is difficult to consistently maintain a positive outlook and feelings of gratitude. If, however, we accept that every circumstance has a meaning for our lives and is therefore a learning experience, expressing thankfulness becomes easier. Adopt the attitude that there is no good or bad, because no matter the circumstances, everything is an arrangement of God.

Remember to continuously congratulate yourself on all successes, whether large or small, and acknowledge that you are on your way to permanent weight loss.

> Remember to continuously congratulate yourself on all successes, whether large or small.

4

Research and Discussion

Good Fats

Contrary to popular belief, eating fat will not necessarily make you fat. In fact, a certain type will actually help you *lose* fat.

Two essential fatty acids, omega-3 and omega-6, are polyunsaturated fats but called by many as good (omega-3) and bad (omega-6) fats. Both of them are "essential" because they are not manufactured by the body and therefore must be eaten in foods. Those who label fatty acids as good or bad don't understand their roles. Along with omega-3 fatty acids, omega-6 fatty acids are crucial for brain health, hair growth, vascular and skin health, and other vital functions of the body.

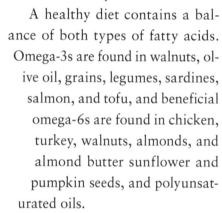

A healthy diet contains a balance of both types of fatty acids. Omega-3s are found in walnuts, olive oil, grains, legumes, sardines, salmon, and tofu, and beneficial omega-6s are found in chicken, turkey, walnuts, almonds, and almond butter sunflower and pumpkin seeds, and polyunsaturated oils.

Omega-6 fatty acids have gotten a bad rap because people in the United States eat many processed and fast foods, such as burgers and fries, that contain large amounts of that fatty acid, creating an imbalance in the body and leading to health issues, including inflammation. By limiting these foods, you will enjoy better physical and mental health.

According to the Mayo Clinic, the Mediterranean diet (low in saturated fat and high in omega-3 fats) reduces the risk of heart disease. The Clinic acknowledges that foods such as olives and olive oil, vegetables, fruit, beans, nuts, whole grains, and even red wine are also important contributors to the diet's benefits.

Egg yolks, organ meats, fatty red meats, farm-raised salmon, turkey, pork, and chicken contain a fat known as arachidonic acid. Consumed in moderation, arachidonic acid is an important source of nutrition, but too much of it can harm the body and cause inflammation. To avoid health risk with foods that contain arachidonic acid, balance them with the omega-3 foods listed above. The Mediterranean diet has limited arachidonic acid.

Creating a Vision

Frankly, I don't like to exercise. It takes time and I find it boring. In the past, I exercised only to stay healthy and toned. But after watching eighty-three-year-old Cloris Leachman on the television program *Dancing with the Stars*, I became inspired to exercise with enthusiasm.

Anyone who has seen the competition on *Dancing with the Stars* knows that to perform at such a level, the dancers must practice hours every day. Competitive ballroom dancing requires great stamina and tremendous motivation. Not only was Ms. Leachman up to the task, but she was also spectacular!

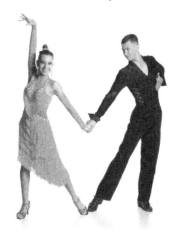

I asked myself if I, a much younger senior than Ms. Leachman, could dance like her. And the answer was a resounding no.

But my imagination started getting the better of me. I pictured myself on the show, wearing a revealing costume with a bare waist and dancing my heart

4

Create the body you want by sculpting a vision in your mind.

out. Surely, if an eighty-three-year-old woman can do this, I can. This inspiration has helped me maintain a regular exercise routine for the last few years. Whenever I hesitate to go to the fitness center or start to get bored exercising, I remember my vision.

One day, I suddenly had the idea to do some arm exercises along with aerobic jogging, and now they have become part of my routine. In just over a month, I was amazed by how many inches I had lost from my waist and upper hip area. It may seem like a coincidence that I started exercising regularly and that I thought to add the arm exercises to my program, but believe me, it is not a coincidence.

My mind embraced the vision of my dancing for a huge audience on network television and, as a result, provided the information and motivation to make my vision a reality. (I am delighted that my figure continues to shape up to match my mind's image.)

Keep an eye out for me on *Dancing with the Stars* sometime in the future! I'll be wearing that revealing little number and performing previously impossible gyrations.

(Since creating this personal vision, I was selected to dance in Japan with a group of sixty people from North America. Ten thousand people from around the world attended a special ceremony and watched as our group represented our continent in an artistic presentation. Perhaps this is my *Dancing with the Stars*.)

If I can do it, so can you. Create the body you want by sculpting a vision in your mind.

Theory of the Mind

You decided to be overweight before your teenage years!

I can imagine your confusion as you unsuccessfully try to recall the time you made this decision. After much thought, most of you will conclude, "It never happened." Well, it did happen.

Most of your personality traits, behaviors, and habits are the

Margianna Langston

4

result of positive or negative subconscious decisions you made before puberty. A better understanding of how you made those decisions can strengthen your faith in this program.

The child's mind starts very early to put together a script that dictates personality, behaviors, hopes, fears, and beliefs. Newborns are open books with no preconceived ideas. As they grow and gain life experience, they begin to absorb information that forms beliefs.

Unfortunately, what children take into their minds doesn't always follow any logic. They often misinterpret information, accepting it as fact (and those "facts" become their truths). Through this development process, children become success-oriented or failure-oriented, depending on the input they receive. They evolve as they construct themselves, deciding their self-worth and establishing confidence (or a lack thereof).

When you sow a seed for a tomato plant, you expect it to produce tomatoes. Likewise, adults will harvest whatever seeds have been planted in their subconscious minds as children.

Noted marriage and family counselor and hypnotherapist Dr. John Kappas taught that our brain power is divided approximately as follows (see the diagram on page 62):

- Conscious mind: 10 to 12 percent

- Subconscious mind: 80 to 85 percent

- Genetic predisposition: 5 to 10 percent

When infants are held, fed, and diapered, their perception is "I am loved." In this instance, the subconscious mind makes a positive decision that lays the foundation for the child's development. Neglected babies would have the opposite perception and make a negative decision about their self-worth. Many studies indicate that unloved babies are often damaged psychologically and may be slow to develop physically.

4

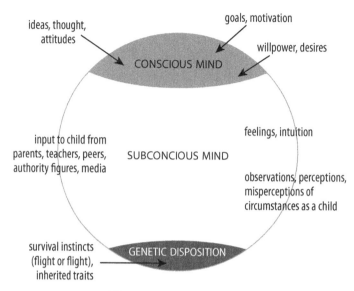

Theory of the Mind

For good or bad, the child's mind remains open and malleable and is constantly accepting input. We have often heard parents utter, "My child misses nothing," or "Little pitchers have big ears."

It is true that children's minds are like sponges, absorbing everything they hear, feel, see, perceive, and so on. They sort and analyze external and internal input and perceive it as truth.

These truths, often distorted by the immature mind, can lead to decisions that adversely affect the happiness of children when they become adults. After the age of twelve or thirteen, the possibility of changing basic characteristics becomes more difficult.

Weight Loss and Theory of the Mind

Suppose that on January 1, you decide to lose twenty pounds. With great excitement and resolve, you begin exercising and eating less. And, by golly, the weight magically begins to disappear.

After three months, you can celebrate because you now fit

into that smaller size bathing suit. The diet is over. As you return to eating normally, you notice that the weight gradually begins to reappear.

You say, "I'm eating too much" or "My metabolism has slowed" or "My family genes have kicked in."

While all these statements may be true, they are not the cause of your weight gain. The cause stems from your subconscious belief system, which is convinced that you will always be twenty pounds overweight. You are fulfilling the expectations of your subconscious.

When you look back at the diagram on page 62, notice that willpower and goals are conscious choices. However, the subconscious mind, primarily established by the time we are twelve years old, makes up the majority of our mind power. Consequently, it has an overwhelming (and controlling) influence on behavior and outcomes in our lives.

In essence, when we set a conscious goal—"I'm going to lose twenty pounds"—we create a tug-of-war between conscious and subconscious control. It is as though you have ten people on one side in a tug-of-war taking on a team of eighty on the other. It's no contest! The eighty-person team (the subconscious programming team) will inevitably win. But this is not always bad news.

If input from your childhood has led to the decision that "I have a beautiful body" or "I don't gain weight," you won't have a weight problem. On the other hand, you can safely assume that if you do have a problem, your programming is inconsistent with maintaining an ideal weight. It will be incumbent upon you to change that programming so it aligns with your goals.

Genetic Predisposition

Let's look at the role that genetic predisposition plays in our makeup. The newborn infant is placed in the mother's arms, arriving with certain predetermined traits, tendencies, and physical

4

When we set a conscious goal, we create a tug-of-war between conscious and sub-conscious control.

4

characteristics that might influence health (or sickness), physical appearance, and even emotional baggage.

For example, the genes and physical appearance of an individual with red hair, a heart-shaped face, five-foot-five-inch height, and a pug nose will more than likely be similar among close family members.

Still, some aspects of our genetic appearance can be altered. For instance, inherited genes may influence the age when wrinkles begin to appear on the face and body. But nutrition, exercise, and the use of certain skin products can delay the natural

Change Your Mind
Change Your Life

You can blame your weight on your childhood!

As you were growing up, your perceptions and misperceptions came from your observations and from the actions and words of your parents, teachers, or other authority figures, as well as from your own internal feelings.

With each passing year, you reinforce your beliefs with your thoughts or words (for example, "I can't lose weight no matter what I do"). You live up to the identity you created for yourself by overeating, leading a sedentary lifestyle, or continuing other behaviors that have a direct bearing on your current weight.

As you practice each step in the *Unleash the Thin Within* program, you are systematically replacing the erroneous messages about weight that you accepted beginning in childhood.

4

aging process. Therefore, physical appearance is not entirely determined at birth.

What is not obvious is how little of our personality, behaviors, and internal psychological programming can be attributed to genetics. Many people strongly believe that they are powerless to change certain characteristics, including the ability to control their weight, because of their family history. As a self-fulfilling prophecy, this becomes their reality and they have become a victim of their thinking.

You may argue, "You don't understand—being overweight runs in my family."

Don't you believe it!

It may be true that several members of your family are overweight. All of you may have metabolisms that function at the speed of turtles or have an excess of "fat" genes. You, however, do not have to accept and embrace your metabolism—or your genetics. My experience is that physiology and chemistry can be changed.

Seeds of Goodness Everywhere

If every circumstance in life has a purpose, we should learn to dispense with the judgment that a particular situation is bad. Instead, teach yourself to automatically recognize that every incident in life carries seeds of good within it. Whatever is unfolding at this moment is advancing you on your life's path.

For me, situations I initially judged as bad turned out to be the impetus for good. In hindsight, the bad (that was really good) took me to a better place or righted my course. When you catch yourself complaining, stop and express gratitude instead.

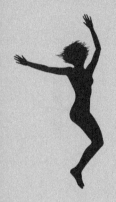

Starting to Thrive 5

The thyroid gland is a relatively small organ located in the lower front of the neck below the larynx. It produces hormones that help control the metabolism, a series of processes by which food is converted into the energy and products needed to sustain life. An underactive thyroid can cause weight gain, fatigue, and depression.

You can strengthen your thyroid by stimulating it yourself. Once you learn this simple technique, you'll be equipped to not only improve your physical health, but also raise your spirits and motivation—the same benefits you can enjoy by regularly lending a hand to others. Add a mind exercise to the mix and you're well on your way to the next level of your holistic journey.

An under-active thyroid can cause weight gain, fatigue, and depression.

Take Action

5.1 **Review Level 4**

5.2 **Determine Your Thyroid Health**
The morning temperature test (performed at home) is a more accurate assessment of thyroid function than measurements of

Margianna Langston

the thyroid hormones in blood tests. An underarm basal (resting) temperature of 97.8°F (36.6°C) or below is considered highly indicative of hypothyroidism (an underactive thyroid), especially when other hypothyroid symptoms are present. Oral temperatures do not correlate closely with thyroid function.

Take your temperature according to the following instructions. Women who menstruate should take their temperature on the second, third, and fourth days of their menstrual period. All others can begin taking their temperature at any time.

- Shake down a basal thermometer at bedtime and place it on a nightstand within easy reach.

- In the morning, before getting out of bed (and without making any unnecessary movement), place the thermometer deep in your left armpit and close your arm firmly on it.

- Leave the thermometer undisturbed inside your armpit for ten minutes. (If you are using a digital thermometer, the button must be pressed at the ten-minute mark.)

- Record your temperature and then resume your daily activities.

- Repeat this temperature test for three to five consecutive mornings. If you record temperatures below normal (97.8), you might want to discuss this finding with your physician and consider nutritional support for enhancing your body's thyroid function.

5.3 Boost Your Thyroid and Metabolism

Stimulate the following applied kinesiology points to enhance thyroid function:

5

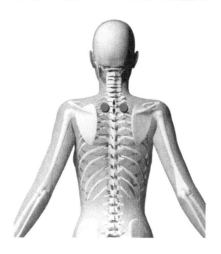

- On the back, massage between the T2 and T3 vertebrae, one inch to each side of the spine.

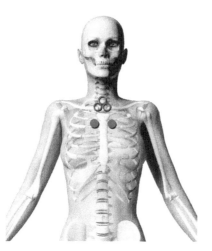

- On the front, massage between the second and third rib on both sides of the breastbone.

- Place three fingers on the depression just above the collarbones while simultaeneously placing a finger on the temple (see below). Hold until a pulse is felt.

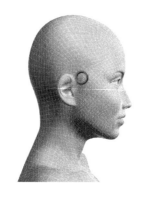

- Place one finger on the temple at the hairline, slightly above and to the front of the ear, while simultaenously placing three fingers on the depression above the breastbone.

5

5.4 Eat Antioxidant-Rich Foods with Every Meal

Antioxidants keep cells healthy so weight gain does not occur. Good sources of antioxidants include many spices, berries, beans, deeply pigmented fruit, dried fruit, herbs, and some vegetables. Here is a partial list of antioxidant- rich foods:

- Beans: black beans, kidney beans, small red beans

- Berries: blueberries, blackberries, raspberries, strawberries

- Other fruits: cantaloupe, mangos, watermelon, plums, cherries, figs

- Nuts and seeds: pecans, walnuts, hazelnuts, pistachio, almonds, cashew nuts, macadamia nuts, peanut butter

- Vegetables: artichokes, broccoli, cabbage, avocados, asparagus, beetroot, spinach, bell peppers, butternut squash

- Spices: clove, cinnamon, turmeric, ginger, garlic, onion, parsley, chili powder, paprika

- Herbs: sage, thyme, marjoram, tarragon, peppermint, oregano, savory, basil, dill weed

5.5 Give to Others

Call, write, or email a family member or friend at least once a week to encourage them or give them your positive input. Research shows that providing emotional support to other people will enhance your own health (even more than receiving help) and help you live longer.

Lending a helping hand to others will make your own life more meaningful while improving your self-image and boosting your motivation to achieve goals (such as weight loss).

> Providing emotional support to other people will enhance your own health and help you live longer.

5

5.6 Walk Mindfully

To continue reprogramming your brain to support permanent weight loss, walk faster than you normally do in all your activities while repeating the affirmation below that has meaning to you. This is similar to the drinking-water exercise on page 41:

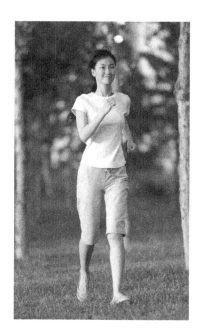

- "With each step I take, I visualize the excess fat in my cells disappearing from my body."

- "With each step I take, I hear the sound of my excess fat breaking off and swiftly moving out of my body."

- "With each step I take, I feel the excess fat dissolving and leaving my body."

Research and Discussion

The thyroid gland is considered a vascular organ, and if its circulation is impaired, it will not get the necessary oxygen and nutrients from the blood to be healthy.

The thyroid gland is stimulated by a hormone from the pituitary gland, and in turn, the thyroid produces hormones that regulate metabolism in every cell of the body. Therefore, potentially all body systems could be affected if the gland isn't functioning properly. Doctors prescribe natural or synthetic hormones for patients with low thyroid hormone levels to return the body to normal.

5

Low Thyroid Function

The following symptoms are associated with an underactive thyroid:

- Weight gain

- Dry skin and hair

- Constipation

- Headaches

- Elevated cholesterol and triglyceride levels

- Paper-thin fingernails

- Swelling of tissues

- Heavy menstrual bleeding

- Weakness

- Fatigue

- Difficulty concentrating

- Forgetfulness

- Depression

If you are experiencing some or all of these symptoms, see your doctor for a complete evaluation of your thyroid. Diagnosing thyroid disease is an involved process that can include clinical evaluation, blood tests, imaging tests, biopsies, and other tests. The good news is that the disease is treatable.

At your appointment, the doctor may . . .

- Weigh you

- Feel your neck (also known as "palpating")

5

- Listen to your thyroid with a stethoscope

- Test your reflexes

- Check your heart rate and rhythm and blood pressure

- Take your temperature

- Examine your face, eyes, hair, skin, nails, and hands

- Order thyroid hormone blood tests

- Order thyroid imaging tests (MRI, CT scan)

Improving Thyroid Health

Nutritionists and other healthcare practitioners advocate a number of ways to improve thyroid gland health, including incorporating the following into your diet and regular practices:

- **Foods with iodine and potassium.** Iodine and potassium are necessary for the health of the thyroid and can be obtained from food sources rather than supplementation unless prescribed by your doctor.

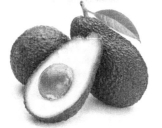

Good sources of iodine include toxin-free sea vegetables, milk, fish, shellfish, and spirulina. Foods rich in potassium are white beans, salmon, dried apricots, dates, bananas, baked acorn squash, baked potatoes, plain yogurt, and avocados. Powdered "greens" are concentrated foods ground into a powder and contain iodine, potassium, and many other minerals, depending on the particular product.

- **Thyroid glandular foods.** The thyroid gland of a cow or pig is an effective nutritional source for rebuilding and repairing the thyroid. These natural foods contain the same vitamins, minerals, amino acids, enzymes and other nutrients found in the human thyroid.

- **Exercise and slant board.** Blood flow to the thyroid can be improved by exercising, lying on a slant board with your legs and feet elevated higher than your head, and standing on your head.

- **Applied kinesiology.** Dr. George Goodheart developed the body of knowledge that came to be known as applied kinesiology. This diagnosis method uses muscle testing as a biofeedback mechanism for determining the energy of organs, glands, and systems. Deficiencies are then corrected by stimulating vascular, lymphatic, and acupressure points, thus restoring the energy flow in the body. For instance, resting your chin lightly on your chest will stimulate your thyroid. See step 5.3 for more exercises.

  Restoring your thyroid's health requires an extended effort. It is not simply a matter of taking a pill and feeling better in the morning. It should become part of an improved nutrition program.

  Always consult your doctor about your thyroid health and follow his or her advice.

Weight Gain and Aging

Free radicals are organic molecules produced when our cells use oxygen and when our body is under attack by unhealthy behaviors. Both actions can damage the tissues and diminish our ability to utilize food efficiently, resulting in a slower metabolism, increased fat storage, and weight gain. While this scenario describes part of the naturally occurring aging process, you can

5

Restoring your thyroid's health is not simply a matter of taking a pill and feeling better in the morning.

5

protect your body by regularly eating antioxidant foods that neutralize free radicals.

Antioxidants can help repair the oxidative damage that can lead to such health problems as heart disease, macular degeneration, diabetes, and cancer. They can also ameliorate the effects of poor food choices, stress, smoking, sun exposure, nutrient deficiencies, and environmental pollution. Five daily servings of fruits and vegetables can significantly reduce health risks by enhancing immune defense.

Margianna Langston

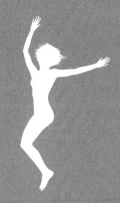

6 Time for a Fix

Life was never meant to be a struggle, but many of us have the mentality that equates achieving goals and success with pain. Some people adopt the mantra "No pain, no gain." It's time to erase that from your mind. Reaching your goals and achieving success in life do not have to be difficult. Persistence may be necessary, but who said it can't be enjoyable?

The way to fulfillment is to pinpoint what makes you happy and pursue it with determination. Keep your eyes focused on the goal and not the effort. Take pleasure in the journey.

In this level, you will learn about the minor changes you can make in your posture and expression that will lift your mood, as well as about the foods you can incorporate into your diet for optimizing your energy and metabolism.

Be excited about your life. It can be fun and rewarding. Remember, though, that your well-being and happiness are up to you. You are in charge of your emotions, your motivation, and ultimately your life. Accept responsibility and create the life you want. It is much easier to accomplish goals, including losing weight, when you are happy and motivated. Practice being happy on demand.

Become the person you want to be.

6

Take Action

6.1 **Review Level 5**

6.2 **Lighten Up**

Smiling and laughing can improve your health and facilitate goal achievement. Never underestimate the power of humor. It takes away your problems, if only for a few seconds. It alleviates stress and tension, creates bonds with others, and changes the body's chemistry.

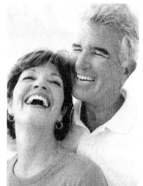

When you look for humor, you will find many opportunities to laugh. The more you laugh, the more you will find things to laugh about. If you don't feel like laughing, fake it (your body doesn't know the difference).

- Laugh consciously at least three times a day.

- Come up with a joke or humorous story to tell your partner each week.

- Perform this laughing exercise: Look in the mirror, stick out your tongue, hold your hands up by your ears, and start laughing as you repeat "Ho, ho, ho, ha, ha, ha, hee, hee, hee." Heartily guffaw for two minutes. Laugh until you are happy.

6.3 **Change Your Body and Change Your Mood**

NLP uses the term "physiology" to refer to posture, facial expressions, and movement. Altering your physiology can have a subtle, but important, influence on the way you feel. It is an easy way to instantly change your mood.

These three exercises can help you experience the effects your physiology has on your emotions and moods:

1. **Bolstering your confidence.**

   - Think of how you would walk, sit, and look if you were extremely confident.

   - Now assume these postures and feel your body chemistry automatically change.

   - Practice these positions throughout the day and stay alert to how they improve your interactions.

2. **Beating the blues.** This is a physical counterpart to the exercise in step 3.4, page 42:

   - Allow yourself to become depressed for several minutes. Notice the body changes that come with depression: slumped shoulders and downcast head and eye.

   - Now, as you continue to feel depressed, sit up with your shoulders thrown back and head and eyes up, with a smile on your face. Then feel depressed. You will find that it's impossible.

   - Practice maintaining a positive posture at least three times a day.

3. **Smiling away negativity.** The mere act of smiling activates a part of the brain that creates pleasure. Smiling on a consistent basis establishes a habit of feeling good, positive, and full of life.

   - Every day after you get up and then before you go

6

to bed, look in the mirror and smile (even grin) at yourself for several minutes.

- Like me, you may feel so foolish that you begin laughing, creating even more positive energy while stimulating the immune system.

- Perhaps you think this is too simple to work? Try it and judge for yourself.

Change your physiology and change your life!

6.4 Consume Metabolism-Beneficial Foods and Beverages

- **Water.** Recent research indicates that drinking water actually speeds up weight loss.

- **Green tea.** Green tea extracts boost metabolism and may aid in weight loss. This mood-enhancing tea has also been reported to contain anti-cancer properties and help prevent heart disease.

- **Soup.** Eat less and burn fat faster by having a bowl of soup as an appetizer or a snack. According to a Penn State University study, soup is a super appetite suppressant because it's made up of a hunger-satisfying combination of liquids and solids.

- **Grapefruit.** Researchers at Scripps Clinic found that the unique chemical properties in vitamin C–packed grapefruit reduces insulin levels, thereby promoting weight loss and boosting metabolism. *Note*: If you are taking medication, check with your doctor about any potentially adverse interactions with this citrus fruit.

- **Broccoli.** Studies have linked calcium and weight loss. Broccoli is high in calcium as well as vitamin C, which increases calcium

6

absorption. In addition to fighting fat, this weight-loss superfood contains powerful phytochemicals that enhance your immunity and protect against disease.

- **High-protein foods (lean meat, fish, poultry, tofu).** Countless studies indicate that protein can help increase metabolism, lose fat, and build lean muscle tissue so you burn more calories.

- **High-fiber foods.** Oatmeal, barley, and wheat bran are good sources of fiber. Steel cut or rolled oats are also heart healthy because they can reduce cholesterol and are fat-soluble, creating a feeling of fullness and providing energy.

More Metabolism Boosters

- Calcium

- Berries

- Oily fish

- Extra virgin olive oil

- Low-sugar cereal or grains

- Almonds (one ounce) and peanut butter or almond butter (one tablespoon)

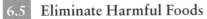

6.5 **Eliminate Harmful Foods**

Work to cut back and then completely remove these foods from your diet:

- **Caffeine.** Found in coffee, tea, and colas, caffeine stimulates the central nervous system. In large amounts, it can cause nervous-

6

ness, irritability, insomnia, tremors, increased heart stimulation, and depression. Caffeine overstimulates and weakens the adrenal glands, eventually resulting in fatigue and possibly creating a negative effect on other hormonal systems. Toxic chemicals are used in growing coffee, and acid in the beans can be harmful to your body as well.

- **Sugar.** Refined sugar is considered to be one of the most harmful foods in our diet. According to the New Hampshire Department of Health and Human Sources, the average American consumes 152 pounds of sugar each year, or three pounds (six cups) of sugar every week. In addition to causing tooth decay, excess sugar consumption can lead to problems with blood sugar levels, thick and sticky blood, adrenal gland exhaustion, and accelerated cellular damage.

- **Artificial sweeteners.** Amounts of potentially dangerous substances, such as lead, arsenic, methanol, and chlorinated disaccharides and monosaccharides, are used to manufacture artificial sweetener products. Ingestion of these chemicals may contribute to serious chronic immunological or neurological disorders.

Research and Discussion

Laughter Is the Best Medicine

In his book *Anatomy of an Illness as Perceived by the Patient*, Norman Cousins relates the story of being diagnosed with ankylosing spondylitis—a degenerative arthritic disorder—and learning that he had little chance of recovery.

Convinced that laughter could improve his condition, he asked his nurse to show him Marx Brothers movies. "I made the joyous discovery that ten minutes of genuine belly laughter

Margianna Langston

had an anesthetic effect and would give me at least two hours of pain-free sleep," he said.

Norman Cousins actively worked to cure himself of an "incurable" illness and was successful. This was revolutionary back in the 1960s and remains so even today.

Subsequent studies have proven the correlation between laughter and enhanced immune cell function. The benefits of laughter can affect every system in the body, including the following:

- Cardiovascular

- Respiratory

- Muscular

- Central nervous

- Endocrine

Research has shown that laughter provides these health benefits:

- **Improved blood flow.** Blood vessels more easily expand and contract.

- **Stronger immune response.** The level of infection-fighting antibodies and immune cells rises.

- **Lower blood sugar levels.** Diabetics experience a decrease in blood sugar.

- **Better sleep.** Relaxation and sleep is enhanced.

Smiling and laughing will reportedly help you fight off colds and flu, diseases, and type 2 diabetes. Research has shown that not only can laughter reduce food cravings, but it can also increase the metabolism by 10 to 20 percent—two more excellent

6

Smiling and laughing will reportedly help you fight off colds and flu, diseases, and type 2 diabetes.

6

reasons to laugh a lot! There is even an emerging field known as humor therapy that can help people heal more quickly.

No drug or pill can provide the same benefits as a positive outlook. And the healthier you are, the more positive you can be and the better you can focus on your goals and sustain the motivation needed to succeed.

So smile and express gratitude for all you are, all you have, and all God has created. Laugh heartily and often.

> No drug or pill can provide the same benefits as a positive outlook.

Smile

Smiling is infectious,
you catch it like the flu.
When someone smiled at
    me today,
I started smiling too.

I passed around the corner,
and someone saw my grin.
When he smiled I realized,
I'd passed it on to him.

I thought about that smile,
then I realized its worth.
A single smile just like mine,
could travel the earth.

So, if you feel a smile begin,
don't leave it undetected.
Let's start an epidemic
    quick,
and get the world infected!

—Karen
McLendon-Laumann

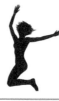

Laughing Away the Pounds

Here are three jokes to get you started on your journey to health through laughter:

For those of you who watch what you eat, here is the final word on nutrition and health. It's a relief to know the truth after all those conflicting medical studies. The Japanese eat very little fat and suffer fewer heart attacks than Americans. The Mexicans eat a lot of fat and suffer fewer heart attacks than Americans. The Chinese drink very little red wine and suffer fewer heart attacks than

6

Americans. The Italians drink large amounts of red wine and suffer fewer heart attacks than Americans. Conclusion: Eat and drink what you like—speaking English is apparently what kills you!

Three friends from the local congregation were asked, "When you're in your casket, and friends and congregation members are mourning over you, what would you like them to say?"

Artie said, "I would like them to say I was a wonderful husband, a fine spiritual leader, and a great family man."

Eugene commented, "I would like them to say I was a wonderful teacher and servant of God who made a huge difference in people's lives."

Al said, "I'd like them to say, 'Look, he's moving!'"

Smith climbs to the top of Mt. Sinai to get close enough to talk to God.

Looking up, he asks, "God, what does a million years mean to you?"

God replies, "A minute."

Smith asks, "And what does a million dollars mean to you?"

God replies, "A penny."

Smith asks, "Can I have a penny?"

God replies, "In a minute."

Foods That Support Weight Loss

Learning more about different foods and choosing them wisely will help you block, burn, or fight fat.

- **Fat blockers.** Foods in the fat-blocker category sit at the top of the fullness scale. They have high-fiber content and satisfy hunger without excess amounts of fat and calories. Fiber and high-bulk foods move slowly through the digestive tract, providing a

6

lasting source of metabolic fuel and lessening your food cravings. Consume them in the morning or early afternoon:

- Oat or wheat bran
- Apples and pears
- Berries
- Leafy greens and other vegetables

- **Fat burners.** Fat burners create thermal energy within the body, boosting metabolism and helping you to actually burn calories while eating. They are mostly high-protein foods:

  - Eggs
  - Lean beef steak
  - Fish
  - Extra lean ground beef
  - Poultry
  - Peanut butter
  - Tofu
  - Vegetarian meat substitutes
  - Cayenne pepper
  - Chromium

- **Fat fighters.** An important fat fighter is chromium. It builds lean tissue and encourages the body to focus on burning fat rather than muscle when energy is needed. Chromium also helps the thyroid function efficiently, boosts the basal metabolic rate, and assists in normalizing insulin levels.

6

Excellent sources of chromium are romaine lettuce, onions, and tomatoes, along with brewer's yeast, oysters, liver, whole grains, bran cereals, and potatoes.

The Science of Metabolism Boosters

Use the following information to guide your food choices:

- **Calcium.** A University of Tennessee study found that dieters who consumed between 1,200 and 1,300 milligrams (mg) of calcium a day lost nearly twice as much weight as dieters getting less calcium. The calcium in milk is a metabolic trigger.

- **Jalapeno and cayenne peppers.** Capsaicin is the chemical in hot peppers that definitely gives them their heat, and it may fire up the metabolism too. Disagreement exists among scientists about whether peppers in the diet make a significant difference in weight loss if they are not combined with other metabolic boosters. One study shows that eating a spicy meal can raise the metabolism by up to 25 percent, with increased burning of calories lasting up to three hours after eating. Another study reports that the metabolism is not affected by spices at all.

- **Protein.** Thermic effect is the measure by which the metabolism increases when stimulated. Protein has a greater thermic effect than carbohydrates and fats, so it's important to eat protein with each meal. Exercise also creates a thermic effect.

- **Green tea.** Green or white tea is rich in antioxidants that prevent and repair cellular damage. A recent study found that subjects who took green tea extract burned an average of 4 percent more calories over the course of a day. Although green tea has caffeine, it does not affect the body detrimentally as other caffeinated drinks do.

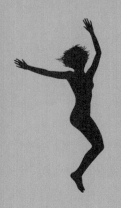

Metabolism Game Changers 7

Metabolism is the sum total of all the processes the body needs to function, including the breakdown of proteins, carbohydrates, and fats to yield vital energy. When these processes are sluggish or inefficient, so is the metabolism. Causes of this suboptimal condition include chronic constipation, lack of exercise, insomnia, poor food choices, and hot or cold air temperatures.

> A strong digestive system is one of the key components for achieving optimal health.

Take Action

7.1 **Review Level 6**

7.2 **Eliminate Chronic Constipation**
A strong digestive system is one of the key components for achieving optimal health. If you are constipated, it is important to resolve it so you can achieve your weight-loss goals.

When the digestive system does not work efficiently and constipation occurs, the transfer and absorption of essential nutrients into the body is impaired. Food waste remains in the intestines for prolonged periods and toxins build up when we

Margianna Langston

7

can't eliminate them through regular bowel movements. Constipation is usually caused by a problem with the bowel function, such as a nerve or muscle disorder, rather than with its structure.

The best way to avoid waste buildup in the body is to eat a supportive diet that includes food with high-fiber content, such as fresh fruits, leafy green vegetables, whole grains, legumes, nuts, and seeds. Apples and beets are natural laxatives.

Also, drink plenty of fluids. When your body is deprived of the water it needs to regularly flush out your system, waste accumulates and hardens in the intestines, causing constipation. Drinking sixty-four ounces of water every day is commonly recommended as a healthful practice for everyone. But it should be water, not coffee, tea, soda, or alcohol, because they may actually exacerbate dehydration and bring on constipation.

Always keep a container of fresh, clean water within reach.

7.3 Be Cool

Keep your indoor temperature cool and exercise outdoors in cold weather whenever possible. Your body will burn more calories as it works to keep you warm.

7.4 Get Plenty of Z's

Studies report that insufficient sleep can have significant harmful effects on a person's health and might even affect weight.

When we sleep, our bodies take care of basic body maintenance tasks, including pumping blood, breathing, and repairing damaged tissues. A lack of sleep reduces the amount of calories your body burns while resting and can seriously impede weight

7

loss. So make sure you get seven to eight hours of sleep every night.

7.5 Move Your Body

An excellent way to jump-start your metabolism and reduce constipation is with physical activity. Exercise for thirty minutes three to four times a week. It will decrease body fat and increase lean muscle mass. Because muscle tissue metabolizes more calories than fat tissues, your metabolism will increase as your muscle mass increases.

So not only does a muscle-toned body look more appealing, but increased muscle mass also facilitates weight loss. And the benefits of aerobic exercises, such as brisk walking, swimming, or riding a bicycle, last far beyond the activity. Here are exercise guidelines:

- **Time of day.** There is no reliable evidence to suggest that calories are burned more efficiently at certain times of the day. But the time of day can influence how you feel when exercising. The most important thing, experts say, is to choose a time of day you can stick with, so that exercise becomes a habit.

- **Amount.** For the greatest overall health benefits, professionals recommend moderate-intensity aerobic exercise most days of the week and anaerobic exercise, such as muscle-strengthening activity and stretching, at least two or three times a week. A minimum of twenty to thirty minutes of exercise every other day is sufficient to stimulate metabolism and build lean muscle mass.

- **Variety.** Changing an exercise routine on a regular basis will help with motivation. Some experts suggest that the body adapts to exercise and eventually stops adding lean muscle; therefore, the type of exercise you perform should be changed every two to

Not only does a muscle-toned body look more appealing, but increased muscle mass facilitates weight loss.

7

three weeks. Other experts disagree. What is most important is to consistently perform exercise you enjoy, whether it's walking, jogging, tennis, or weight-lifting so you will continue doing it.

Research and Discussion

A Happy, Healthy Colon

Dr. Mehmet Oz and others advocate cleaning the colon to aid weight-loss efforts. Numerous options are available to remove harmful toxins and waste that accumulate in the intestines. Some people go to a healthcare professional for colon therapy, an infusion of water into the rectum that washes out the colon. Trapped waste can be eliminated in this way.

While many laxatives, including herbal products, are widely available in drug stores, grocery stores, health food stores, and other retail distribution outlets, they should be used with care. They may relieve constipation, but they may endanger your health in other ways, such as:

- Killing friendly (necessary) intestinal bacteria

- Diminishing your body's absorption of nutrients and vitamins

- Risking dependence

If you take a laxative on occasion, be sure to eat low- or no-sugar yogurt or kefir to help regain your intestinal bacteria balance.

Note: If you take certain medications or over-the-counter drugs that have constipating side effects, be sure to talk to your physician about healthier alternatives. Never stop taking prescribed medications without the consent and supervision of your doctor.

7

Causes of Constipation

Foods causing constipation:

- Processed foods: white bread, instant mashed potatoes, white rice, and white pasta

- Bananas

- Caffeine (because of its dehydrating effect)

- Dairy products

- Chocolate

Other causes of constipation:

- Lack of exercise and a sedentary lifestyle

- Low-fiber diet

- An insufficient amount of fluid intake

- Over-the-counter medications—overuse of laxatives and antacids containing calcium or aluminum

- Insufficient digestive enzymes produced by the pancreas

- Lack of certain kinds of fat in the diet

- Food allergies

The Role of Exercise

A sedentary lifestyle is quite literally constipating. Exercise brings more blood, oxygen, and nutrients to the intestines to support proper functioning, and when combined with recommended dietary changes, it will aid your body's ability to keep your colon clean, reducing instances of constipation.

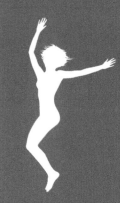

8 Positively Vibrate and Model Success

We respond to the vibrations that our thoughts create. If we think that we will never reach a particular goal, our failure will be assured.

> *Watch your thoughts, they become your words. Watch your words, they become your actions. Watch your actions, they become your habits. Watch your habits, they become your character. Watch your character, it becomes your destiny.*
>
> (Author unknown—the passage has been attributed to many people throughout the years.)

Take Action

8.1 **Review Level 7**

8.2 **Immerse Yourself in Positive Thoughts**
It is important to surround yourself with positive people who encourage you to accomplish your goals. Think about everyone in your life:

8

Thoughts hold the power to create.

- List the people closest to you.

- Review the list to determine if these people are upbeat and supportive.

- If you perceive them as negative, ask them to think and speak in a positive way about your program goals. Or don't discuss your weight-loss program with them.

Your thoughts have vibrations and vibrations create energy. *Thoughts hold the power to create.*

Idle thoughts accumulate over time. If positive, they will support your success, but if negative, they can eventually drown you in discouragement and failure. The following exercise demonstrates how much our thoughts affect our body and emotions:

First, think of a negative event in your life (a thoroughly unpleasant experience). As you recall it, notice what happens within your body and with your emotions.

- Do you feel anger, resentment, or another negative emotion?

- Does tension fill your body? Do you feel your neck and shoulders becoming tight?

- Do you feel irritable, impatient, or even hostile?

Next, imagine your favorite place in nature. Where is it? Is it a beach, a mountain top, or the woods? As you feel the sun on your face and smell the fresh air, notice your body's response.

- Do you feel peaceful and happy?

- Does your body relax?

The linkage between our thoughts and feelings is a compel-

8

ling argument for learning to catch negative thoughts as they arise and to put a positive spin on every situation. Always find the silver lining.

Practice this exercise daily over the next three weeks: Be conscious of when you have a negative thought and immediately change it to a positive one or to gratitude. You can easily do this by remembering a time when you were happy and feeling on top of the world or by thinking of something you're grateful for. If you do this with sincerity, it will be impossible to be negative.

Also, when you have a negative thought or get upset or disturbed by a situation, say to yourself, "So what." This reminds you not to sweat the small stuff.

8.3 Establish a Relaxation Anchor

High on the list of fears is public speaking. An estimated three out of every four people experience some degree of anxiety when speaking before an audience. If you fit this description—or if you have other fears—the following steps can help you create a positive anchor (trigger) that will relax your mind and body:

- Think of an occasion when you had a highly pleasurable, memorable, and relaxing experience.

- Visualize this scene in great detail and vivid color.

- Hear what you heard at that time—perhaps birds singing or someone speaking loving words about you.

- Feel what you felt, such as totally loved, successful, joyful, or amused.

- Create a movie in your mind of this pleasant occasion. Remember your thoughts, conversations, and strong relaxation or pleasurable feelings as you star in this movie.

8

- As your memory re-creates the sensations you experienced, allow them to increase in intensity.

- Create an anchor for this memory by touching your left hand gently to your left thigh for several seconds, and then remove your hand.

- Think of something else for a few moments.

- Then once again re-create the memory of that relaxing occasion you thought about moments before.

- Touch your left hand to your left thigh.

- Release this pose.

- Continue replaying the memory of that pleasurable occasion while creating your anchor until you feel relaxed simply by touching your hand to your thigh.

The next time you stand before a group of people to speak and feel nervous or have any other anxiety-provoking experience, activate your anchor by touching your left hand to your left thigh. (No one will notice and you will be amazed at the calmness that comes over your mind and body.)

8.4 Find a Model and Create an Anchor

Think of someone you really admire who has traits you would like to adopt as your own, such as the following:

- Physical attributes

- Mental outlook

- Ability to love and care for others

- Spontaneity

- Happiness

Margianna Langston

8

- Special talent

- Confidence

Complete these steps with your partner and your model's traits will soon become part of you:

- Identify a few specific physical attributes of the person you wish to model, such as posture, gait, and facial expression.

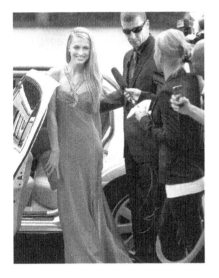

- Carefully observe, study, and practice copying those attributes.

- If the person you chose to model is a celebrity or public figure, read articles or books that describe her upbringing, fitness routine, road to success, and so on. If you know the individual, ask her these same questions. (Don't be shy—she will be flattered!)

- Practice copying the person's posture while your partner observes and helps you adopt her mannerisms. Include small details such as how she holds her hands, tilts her head, and carries her shoulders.

- Notice the way this person talks (pace, pitch, and inflection).

- Think thoughts that you imagine your model would have.

- Practice mimicking your subject, keeping a detailed picture firmly in your mind while creating an anchor.

8

Then, set aside five minutes at bedtime to close your eyes, tap into your imagination, and become your model. Use your senses as you do this:

- Sight: How do you look?

- Sound: What are you saying internally and what is your model saying to you?

- Feeling: What are your emotions?

- Once your mind embraces the image of your model, touch your thumb and forefinger together to create an anchor.

- Practice this exercise in its entirety at bedtime for seven consecutive nights. The image of your model will become clearer and more strongly associated with you as every day passes.

- After seven days, touch your thumb and forefinger together several times a day to activate your anchor. The change you desire becomes more embedded in your subconscious mind every time you do this.

According to numerous studies, optimistic people tend to be healthier and live longer.

Research and Discussion

Norman Vincent Peale's classic book, *The Power of Positive Thinking*, was at the forefront of positive thought psychology when it was published decades ago. Just as relevant today, his message is now backed up by scientific evidence.

According to numerous studies, optimistic people tend to be healthier and live longer. In *The Power of Appreciation* by Dr. Noelle C. Nelson and Dr. Jeannine Lemare Calaba, Dr. Nelson reports, "Appreciation is a dynamic energy force, functioning according to scientific principles. This energy can be harnessed

8

"I'm a Failure"

Notice when you think you have done something "wrong" and put yourself down in your thoughts. Then notice when you do something "right"—what do you say to yourself then? Most people say nothing. Start congratulating yourself for your successes.

Beating yourself up is counterproductive to achieving success. Accept that there is no messing up. Whatever you did or didn't do is now in the past. Learn from it and then put it behind you because it no longer matters.

Concentrate on doing your best and abandon judging yourself. As previously recommended, adopt the attitude that there is no good or bad, because no matter the situation, everything is an arrangement of God.

And if you say you will "try" to change your thinking, you acknowledge the possibility of failure. Remove that limiting word from your vocabulary. Develop a mindset of "I can do it"! As Yoda says, "There is no try, only do."

As you practice these exercises, you will be amazed by how much your life will improve.

by anyone to achieve success, happiness, and fulfillment in every area of life: from finances to work to family to health to aging and even in crisis." The book provides a five-step process to "transform troubling situations and attract successful and joyous experiences."

The authors also say that "appreciation is literally magic for your life." They point to several scientific studies that demon-

8

strate the power this emotion has on our health and well-being. The following MRI scans illustrate the impact that positive thoughts have on brain function:

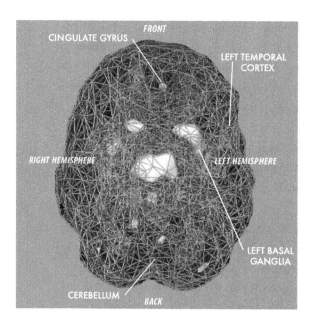

MRI brain scan of the subject having negative thoughts and feelings

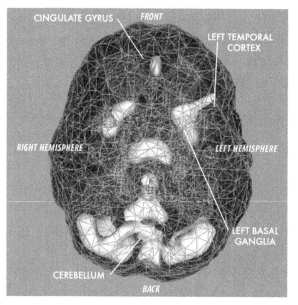

MRI brain scan of the subject having positive thoughts and feelings

Margianna Langston

8

When the subject experienced negative thoughts and feelings, blood flow to the brain decreased. Conversely, when the subject experienced positive thoughts and feelings, blood flow to the brain increased.

The dramatic images captured in the MRI scans show us that changing our thinking to eliminate negative thoughts and sabotaging self-talk is fundamental to our health.

Creating Anchors

NLP anchoring is an effective technique that can help you deliberately change your state of mind. By connecting an anchor (or trigger) to a specific mood—such as peaceful, happy, or enthusiastic—you can immediately move to that mood whenever you activate the anchor, much like Pavlov's conditioning.

You create an NLP anchor by associating a unique visual, auditory, or physical stimulus with a particular emotional state. For example, when you're feeling confident, anchor that feeling to a light pinch with your thumb on your right little finger. Repeat that process numerous times. Once the anchor is conditioned, every time you pinch your right little finger, you will feel confident.

Negative anchors can be inadvertently created by negative circumstances in our lives. For many years, whenever I got a phone call early in the morning, my heart raced, fearful thoughts gripped my mind, and my neck and shoulders tightened instantly. Why? Because when my children were young, I received a call at six o'clock one morning, relaying a message that one of them was in danger. This traumatic experience became imbedded in my mind.

Even though years had gone by, early-morning calls triggered an automatic visceral fear response for me. Only after I neutralized this negative anchor by attaching positive thoughts to it was I able to peacefully accept early calls.

> MRI scans show us that changing our thinking to eliminate negative thoughts is fundamental to our health.

8

Modeling What You Admire

You can supercharge the positive effects of the anchoring technique when you combine anchoring with another powerful NLP and behavioral tool, commonly referred to as modeling.

My friend Sherrie has such beautiful posture and I once asked her how she developed it. She told me that when she would slump over as a child, her mother would whack her between the shoulders to remind her to stand tall.

Since I want to have posture like Sherrie's, I created a special anchor as follows to help me achieve that: I visualize Sherrie and my shoulders automatically lift and my posture improves. I use my mind's image of her as my anchor. As a result, my body responds to the anchor and mimics Sherrie's posture (without anyone whacking me between my shoulders), and she is flattered that I want to be like her in this way.

Model those you admire. Adopt their characteristics, behaviors, and attitudes by creating anchors. By practicing these NLP techniques, you will see improvement in every area of your life that you focus on.

Succeeding

To make significant changes and improvements in your life, remember these three steps:

1. PRACTICE

2. PRACTICE

3. PRACTICE

Be grateful every morning when you wake up and remember that you are moving closer to your goal.

---

9 A Healthy Body Boosts Motivation

An unhealthy body affects the mind (including motivation) and physical abilities. When you have a foggy head and chronic fatigue and generally feel unwell, it is difficult to focus on a goal and take the necessary steps to achieve it.

To successfully complete this program, you must feel good. While it is important to enlist a doctor's help, don't make the mistake of relying solely on medical professionals. Do your part, because your good health depends largely on your behaviors and mindset.

It's important to pay close attention to your adrenal glands, the pair of pea-sized glands located on top of each kidney. An essential part of the endocrine system, these organs release hormones that help us handle stress.

The adrenals can and do burn out from years of battling the repeated onslaught of stressors, such as insufficient sleep, unrelenting fatigue and pain, emotional stress, a bad diet, or reliance on a plethora of prescription medications. The result is chronic poor physical, mental, and emotional health. By adopting the stress-reduction habits ahead, you can make significant improvements in your overall well-being.

The adrenals can and do burn out from years of battling the repeated onslaught of stressors.

9

Take Action

9.1 Review Level 8

9.2 Perform the Adrenal Gland Test

A very simple home test of adrenal function, the Ragland Test, is explained below:

- Relax for ten minutes and take your blood pressure lying down.

- Your partner records your blood pressure.

- Immediately stand up and take your blood pressure again.

- Record your standing blood pressure numbers.

An increase of ten to twenty millimeters in the systolic (top) number is normal. A decrease or failure to increase is abnormal and indicates adrenal fatigue. Upon standing, you may feel weak, slightly dizzy, or shaky.

9.3 Strengthen Your Adrenals

Eliminate or reduce your consumption of these foods:

- Refined sugar products (candy, desserts, and processed snacks)

- Refined carbohydrates (bread, pasta, and rice)

- Caffeine and alcohol

- Processed or junk foods

And add more of the following:

- Nutritious foods in their natural state

- Fiber (whole grains, fruits, vegetables, legumes, nuts, and seeds)

Nutrient-rich foods can supply much of the needed vitamins, minerals, amino acids, enzymes, and fiber that your body needs to repair. They include:

- Dairy products

- Healthy protein (lean beef, fish, chicken, eggs, and tofu)

- Concentrated powdered greens

- Glandular foods

- Bee pollen

- Wheat grass

- Spirulina

The body can select what it needs from the array of nutrients contained within these foods without jeopardizing its natural nutrient balance.

Adrenal exhaustion can lead to hypoglycemia (low blood sugar). For people suffering from severe hypoglycemia, eating the recommended six mini-meals a day will help maintain the blood sugar at normal levels. Individuals with symptoms of hypoglycemia should always have nutritious snacks within easy access and never skip breakfast or other meals.

While certain nutritional supplements can help treat hypoglycemia, if you suspect you have it or any other serious condition such as diabetes (high blood sugar), consult your doctor before taking supplements. Never take medications or supplements before obtaining a medical diagnosis from a licensed physician.

Here are additional dietary guidelines:

9

Adrenal exhaustion can lead to hypoglycemia (low blood sugar).

9

- Eat foods rich in vitamin C, such as citrus fruits and green peppers.

- Avoid drinking large quantities of juices, which are often concentrated carbohydrates, contain refined sugar, and can create blood sugar imbalances in the body.

- Choose whole fruit whenever possible as an alternative to juice; fruits are important sources of fiber.

- Eat foods high in essential oils (salmon, olive oil, flaxseed oil).

- Reduce your consumption of chemicals, which can disrupt your body's functions and make you fat! The average American ingests over one hundred pounds of chemicals (contained in drugs, foods, and beverages) each year. Remember this whenever you consider taking over-the-counter drugs, eating processed foods, or drinking a diet soda.

Stimulate the adrenal glands with applied kinesiology techniques as follows:

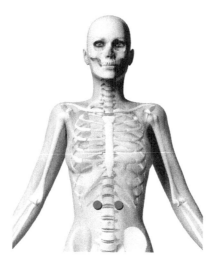

- With circular motion, massage two inches above and one inch to each side of your navel.

9

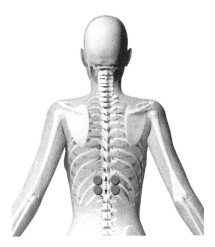

- From the back, massage between the T10-T11 and T11-T12 vertebrae, one inch to each side of the spine, at the last ribs.

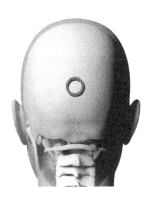

- With two fingers, hold the posterior fontanel (the "soft spot") on the back of the head until a pulse is felt to stimulate blood flow to the adrenal glands.

9.4 Conquer Stress

Identify and reduce your stressors:

- Are you enjoying life?

- Do you stop to smell the roses?

- When was the last time you did something to relax and make yourself happy?

- Simplify your life! What are your values?

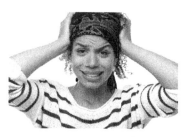

Stress undermines your emotional, mental, and physical health. Emotional stress comes from negative emotions, such as anger, worry, and unhappiness. Mental stress may be caused by your thoughts, conflict with others, indecision, or mental overwhelm. Physical stress can come from temperature extremes, and lack of sleep.

Here are several suggestions for decreasing the stress in your life:

EMOTIONAL STRESS REDUCTION

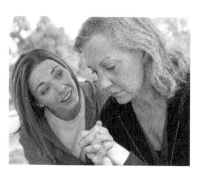

- Share your feelings with a good friend.

- Avoid people who stress you.

- Learn to say no.

- Express feelings instead of bottling them up.

- Reframe your thoughts from negative to positive.

- Revisit step 6 (especially 6.2) for ways to incorporate more laughter and happiness into your life, thereby alleviating tension.

MENTAL STRESS REDUCTION

- Schedule your time and tasks mindfully.

- Relax in a hot bath.

- Stop and breathe deeply:

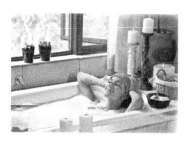

Margianna Langston

9

- Sit in a cross-legged position or lie on your back, on the floor.

- Place one hand on your abdomen and the other on your rib cage.

- Inhale slowly through your nose, allowing your breath to slowly and progressively fill your abdomen, rib cage, upper chest, shoulders, and neck.

- Hold this breath for five seconds.

- Slowly release your breath through your nose.

PHYSICAL STRESS REDUCTION

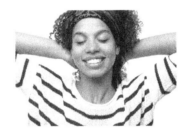

- Sleep seven to eight hours every night.

- Rest when you feel tired.

- Avoid extreme cold or heat.

- Eat nutritious foods that include proteins (chicken, fish, tofu), complex carbohydrates (fruits, vegetables), and unsaturated fats (fatty fish, olive and flax seed oil, nuts, seeds, and avocados).

- Avoid cake, candy, ice cream, syrups, white bread, pasta, and chemical-laden foods.

Research and Discussion

If your mind and body are constantly on edge because of excessive demands in your life, your adrenal glands will constantly release the hormones adrenaline and cortisol. This long-term activation of the stress-response system and the resulting over-

9

exposure to stress hormones can disrupt almost all your body's processes.

Some experts believe that when the adrenal glands are taxed in this way, serious chronic conditions may result, including heart disease, diabetes, hypoglycemia, low or high blood pressure, osteoporosis, compromised immune system, kidney problems, arthritis, and asthma.

Symptoms of adrenal exhaustion include the following:

- Dizziness when standing up

- Low motivation

- Fatigue

- Anxiety

- Decreased mental acuity

- Low body temperature

- Decreased metabolism

Stress and Your Metabolism

Bear in mind that chronic stress will put your body in a constant fight-or-flight mode. When cortisol is released in response, it restricts those functions that would be unnecessary or harmful in a life-threatening situation. Among other actions, cortisol suppresses the digestive system, which in turn slows the metabolism. So reducing stress is also critical to maintaining an efficient metabolism and accomplishing your weight-loss goal.

9

- Depression

- Lowered libido

- Craving for salty foods

- Muscle or joint pains

Adrenal Exhaustion and Low Blood Sugar

As mentioned above, adrenal exhaustion can lead to hypoglycemia, the medical term for low blood sugar. While this condition is often regarded as the opposite of diabetes, many doctors believe that hypoglycemia is actually the precursor to diabetes.

According to the New Hampshire report cited earlier, two hundred years ago, the average American ate only 2 pounds of sugar a year. By 1970, we were each eating 123 pounds of sugar per year. Today, the average American consumes almost 152 pounds of sugar in one year. Our organs and glands become overworked and exhausted trying to continuously normalize blood sugar levels, often resulting in bodily dysfunctions such as hypoglycemia or diabetes.

Hypoglycemia often manifests in nonspecific ways, making the condition difficult to diagnosis. Here are possible symptoms:

- Depression
- Headaches
- Fatigue
- Anxiety
- Insomnia
- Difficulty concentrating
- Shakiness

- Nausea
- Allergies
- Heart palpitations
- Crying spells
- Craving for sweets
- Obesity
- Sexual dysfunction

Many doctors believe that hypoglycemia is actually the precursor to diabetes.

9

Diet plays a key role in the body's ability to regulate blood sugar levels and handle stress.

Blood sugar fluctuates with food ingestion, going up temporarily and then down as the pancreas, liver, and adrenal glands perform their functions to regulate the sugar in the blood. In reactive hypoglycemia, blood sugar levels elevate upon eating and the body overcompensates in its efforts to bring the blood sugar back down, dropping the sugar to very low levels. On rare occasions, hypoglycemia may be caused by a tumor of the pancreas, liver disease, or overdose of insulin.

Glucose Tolerance Test

To medically diagnose hypoglycemia, a glucose tolerance test is performed. It involves the patient drinking glucose (a sugar), and then having his or her blood sugar level tested at scheduled intervals over six hours.

During the test, the technician records blood sugar levels along with symptoms to determine how the body is handling glucose.

Repairing Adrenal Glands

Strengthening, rebuilding, and repairing the pancreas, adrenal glands, and liver are important for controlling or preventing hypoglycemia and diabetes, as well as improving your overall health.

Moderate exercise and weight loss are critical components. The first and most important step is to change the way you eat. Diet plays a key role in the body's ability to regulate blood sugar levels and handle stress. Until you modify your diet, little improvement will occur.

9

The average American's diet reduces the body's ability to counteract stress. Instead of eating nutrient-rich foods, most of us eat an abundance of empty calorie foods that do not support the body's organs, glands, and cells to maintain health and resist stress. These junk foods are devoid of nutrition, but we eat them because they taste good or we've become addicted to them.

Although sometimes necessary, prescription drugs can take a toll on the body's overall health. The chemicals contained in them are stored in the cells of our vital organs, such as the liver. Chronic use can impair the functioning of our organs and glands.

Warning: Do not stop taking prescribed drugs without consulting your doctor. Sudden withdrawal from certain medications can be dangerous.

Implement natural means, such as exercise, good diet, and stress reduction, to regulate body functions whenever possible.

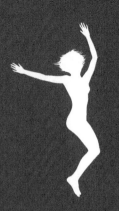

Be Happy, Be Vibrant, Be Alive 10

I do not believe in dieting. But I do believe in eating nutritious foods as a way of life. This may be construed by some as dieting.

If you thought I was subtly (or maybe not so subtly) repeating this belief over and over again throughout this book, you are right. Nourishing foods are essential to your health and well-being and to the success of this spirit, mind, and body approach to weight loss.

If you consider that the body's cells stay healthy when you eat foods containing vitamins, minerals, enzymes, amino acids, and other nutrients, then it makes sense to eat foods that provide such nutrition. This is not dieting but rather a chosen lifestyle that promotes health, energy, and longevity and combats the effects of aging.

And if you recognize that cells are damaged by overdoses of foods with little or no nutrition—refined sugar and white flour products, soft drinks, and chemicals in foods such as monosodium glutamate (MSG), aspartame, preservatives, artificial flavoring, and food colors—it makes sense to reduce or eliminate

Margianna Langston

10

those foods from your diet if you want to be healthy. Eating nutritious foods will not only make you healthy, but also help you reach and maintain your weight-loss goal.

Take Action

10.1 **Review Level 9**

10.2 **Eat for Success**

Eat to stabilize your blood sugar, lose weight, reduce cravings, maintain good health, and increase energy. Here is a summary of the guidelines for selecting the best foods:

PROTEIN (MEAT, FOWL, FISH)

- Limited red meat (beef, lamb, veal) and pork—no more than two servings per week

- Chemical-free meats—read food labels carefully to make sure chemicals such as nitrates have not been added

- Free-range chicken that hasn't been treated with hormones or antibiotics

- Wild fish, without color or other chemicals added

- Canned salmon or sardines—both are inexpensive and good sources of essential fatty acids (good fat) and nutrients

DAIRY PRODUCTS AND EGGS

- Natural cheeses (no synthetic cheeses such as American cheese)—eat in moderation because of its high fat content

10

- Eggs from cage-free chickens (not treated with hormones or antibiotics)

- Yogurt (unsweetened) is loaded with calcium as well as good bacteria that keep your intestines healthy

- Butter in limited quantities

Butter Tip

To reduce the amount of saturated fat in natural butter, prepare it as follows:

- Soften 1 lb. butter at room temperature.

- Mix with ½ to 1 cup olive oil.

- Refrigerate and use as soft butter.

NUTS AND SEEDS

- Almonds
- Walnuts
- Pecans
- Pumpkin seeds

- Brazil nuts
- Pine nuts
- Macadamia nuts
- Sunflower seeds

(*Note:* Peanuts are not recommended.)

VEGETABLES

- Fresh or frozen
- Raw, steamed, or baked

10

- At least one raw salad daily

- Five to eight vegetable servings every day (can be accomplished easily with salads and stir fry dishes) that might include broccoli, kale, spinach, leaf lettuce, beets, cabbage, mushrooms, onions, okra, cauliflower, bok choy, brussels sprouts, celery, parsley, squash, and green beans

- Limited high-carbohydrate vegetables, such as white potatoes, lima beans, corn, and carrots

FRUIT (LOW TO MEDIUM IN COMPLEX SUGARS)

- Berries: blueberries, raspberries, and strawberries

- Watermelon and cantaloupe

- Peaches

- Rhubarb

- Papaya

- Grapefruit

- Apples

- Avocados

BREAD, PASTA, AND CRACKERS

- 100 percent whole wheat, multigrain, or gluten-free breads

- No more than two slices of bread per day

- Whole grain pasta or rice pasta

- Whole grain or rice crackers in limited amounts

10

SPICES

- Herbs are nutritious and add incredible flavor to ordinary dishes.

- Be sure to cook with these healthy herbs: garlic, cayenne, ginger, rosemary, turmeric, and cilantro.

- Stevia is a natural, calorie-free sugar substitute that has no effect on blood sugar.

- Condiments not high in sugar, chemicals, and starch. (Most ketchup, mayonnaise, salad dressing, mustard, relishes, pickles, and sauces contain sugar.)

BEVERAGES

- Water—amount varies according to health and size. Average daily recommendation is eight glasses of eight ounces each (half gallon total); increase water intake for weight loss.

- Lemon water

- Limited low-carbohydrate fruit and vegetable juices: pomegranate, tomato, V-8, cranberry

- Almond and rice milk, kefir (unsweetened)

- Herb teas—green, ginger, astragalus, mint

NO-NOS

- Sugar and products with large amounts of sugar or high fructose corn syrup, including desserts, candies, ketchups, mayonnaise, mustard, salad dressing

- Artificial sweeteners such as sucralose, saccharin, and aspartame

- White bread, white pasta, and white rice

- Vegetables with little nutritional value, such as iceberg lettuce and canned vegetables containing sugar, starch, preservatives, or MSG

- Sodas and caffeine drinks—coffee, strong black tea, energy drinks

- Alcohol

- Meats and chicken with antibiotics or other chemicals

- Farm-raised fish with added color

- Genetically modified soy products

- Artificial foods

Research and Discussion

Make incremental changes to your eating habits over time until you're consuming only nutritious foods. Eventually, you will prefer them to harmful foods because of the new energy and life they bring to you.

Watch your health improve as the following occurs:

- A more alert and creative mind

- A nervous system that says, "Bring it on—I can handle it"

- A body that smiles!

You are capable of reaching your goal—don't sell yourself short. The only thing holding you back is your self-imposed limitations.

Always accept that anything is possible.

10

Always accept that anything is possible.

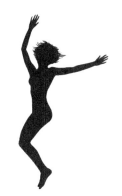

Final Words

Life is a series of choices. In each moment, you can choose your direction, your feelings, your thoughts, your food, your stress level, and ultimately your happiness. For many, this is difficult to accept because it involves letting go of excuses and embracing responsibility for their lives and well-being. Old belief systems often get in the way.

Many people adopt the "I can't change my circumstances" mode. Not true. Circumstances can be changed, although changing ingrained beliefs requires consistent, dedicated effort.

It is important to recognize that *someone* or *something* is not doing anything to you—your actions lead to what become your life experiences. Of course, it is much easier to blame someone else for your stress, lack of self-esteem, lack of success, and unhappiness.

Merely willing something to happen does not automatically shift your mindset so you can create this change: "I accept responsibility for my weight and choose to lose twenty pounds" will not miraculously make you slim. How wonderful if it were that easy.

You now have all the tools you need to be all you choose to

be. The spiritual principles and physical practices and behaviors can be incorporated immediately. Eliminating limiting beliefs, however, is a gradual process. As I emphasized over and over, the secret to success is commitment and persistence. So PRAC-TICE, PRACTICE, and PRACTICE each step and watch with excitement as your body changes.

Appendix A: Success Principles

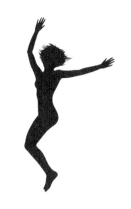

- Hold your dream.

- Sufferings are trainings—through each problem, we can become stronger and grow spiritually, mentally, and physically.

- Gratitude is the key to happiness.

- Self-imposed limitations and resistance sabotage your positive intentions.

- There is no good or bad.

- Listen and observe and you will hear the voice of God.

- The way to success is taking one step at a time.

- Spirit, mind, and body work together, and we must involve all three to create lasting change.

- Everything happens for a purpose—there are no accidents.

- The mind is powerful if harnessed and engaged.

- Focus on what's right in your life, rather than what's wrong or missing.

- Everything you think and say becomes a self-fulfilling prophecy.

- Personal growth is an addiction.

- Let every day be a new beginning and savor each one.

- Lighten up and laugh your way to happiness.

- You can make a difference.

Appendix B: Levels Review

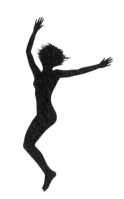

Level 1: Believe, Pray, Commit	Dates Practiced		Date Mastered
	Partner 1	Partner 2	
1. Select a partner			
2. Share your dreams			
3. Make a pact			
4. Discuss your beliefs			
5. Pray for each other daily			
6. Communicate weekly			
7. Cheer each other on			
8. Commit to your goals			
Dates partners talked—in person and over the phone			

Level 2: A Better Way to Eat	Dates Practiced		Date Mastered
	Partner 1	Partner 2	
1. Review level 1			
2. Discuss the commitment passage			
3. Encourage successful outcomes			
4. Increase your metabolism with new eating habits			
Dates partners talked—in person and over the phone			

Level 3: Gratitude Is Key	Dates Practiced		Date Mastered
	Partner 1	Partner 2	
1. Review level 2			
2. Practice gratitude			
3. Adopt an attitude of gratitude for water			
4. Conquer depression			
5. Determine your primary learning style			
Dates partners talked—in person and over the phone			

Level 4: Make Over Your Body and Mind	Dates Practiced		Date Mastered
	Partner 1	Partner 2	
1. Review level 3			
2. Add essential fatty acids (EFAs) to your diet			
3. Savor everything you eat			
4. Change your image			
5. Pat yourself on the back			
Dates partners talked—in person and over the phone			

Level 5: Starting to Thrive	Dates Practiced		Date Mastered
	Partner 1	Partner 2	
1. Review level 4			
2. Determine your thyroid health			
3. Boost your thyroid and metabolism			
4. Eat antioxidant-rich foods with every meal			
5. Give to others			
6. Walk mindfully			
Dates partners talked—in person and over the phone			

Level 6: **Time for a Fix**	Dates Practiced		Date Mastered
	Partner 1	Partner 2	
1. Review level 5			
2. Lighten up			
3. Change your body and change your mood			
4. Consume metabolism-beneficial foods and beverages			
5. Eliminate harmful foods			
Dates partners talked—in person and over the phone			

Level 7: **Metabolism Game Changers**	Dates Practiced		Date Mastered
	Partner 1	Partner 2	
1. Review level 6			
2. Eliminate chronic constipation			
3. Be cool			
4. Get plenty of z's			
5. Move your body			
Dates partners talked—in person and over the phone			

Level 8: Positively Vibrate and Model Success	Dates Practiced		Date Mastered
	Partner 1	Partner 2	
1. Review level 7			
2. Immerse yourself in positive thoughts			
3. Establish a relaxation anchor			
4. Find a model and create an anchor			
Dates partners talked—in person and over the phone			

Level 9: A Healthy Body Boosts Motivation	Dates Practiced		Date Mastered
	Partner 1	Partner 2	
1. Review level 8			
2. Perform the adrenal gland test			
3. Strengthen your adrenals			
4. Conquer stress			
Dates partners talked—in person and over the phone			

Level 10: Be Happy, Be Vibrant, Be Alive	Dates Practiced		Date Mastered
	Partner 1	Partner 2	
1. Review level 9			
2. Eat for success			
Dates partners talked—in person and over the phone			

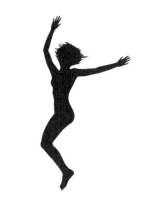

Appendix C: Resources

For further information on the following resources, visit the *Unleash the Thin Within* website: http://unleashthethinwithin.com.

Audio CDs

The Body Ecology *Growing Younger* twelve-disk audio series is an impressive collection of practical information from longevity experts.

Books

The Healing Code: 6 Minutes to Heal the Source of Your Health, Success, or Relationship Issue by Alexander Loyd, PhD, with Ben Johnson, MD. A healing technology for getting and staying well.

The Healing Power of Water by Masaru Emoto. A look at water from the viewpoints of science, healing, and mysticism.

Healing Words: The Power of Prayer and the Practice of Medicine by Larry Dossey, MD. One of the many books Dr. Dossey has written that provides scientific evidence supporting the value of prayer healing.

Mind over Medicine: Scientific Proof That You Can Heal Yourself by Lissa Rankin, MD. A radical new wellness model based on scientific findings.

The Power of Appreciation: The Key to a Vibrant Life by Noelle

C. Nelson, PhD, and Jeannine Lemare Calaba, PsyD. A five-step approach for transforming your life through appreciation.

Touch for Health: A Practical Guide to Natural Health with Acupressure Touch by John Thie, DC, and Matthew Thie, MEd. A comprehensive guide to natural health using acupressure and massage.

Underground Health Reporter: Little-Known Discoveries That Make a Dramatic Impact on Your Health by Think-Outside-the-Book Publishing. A compilation of cutting-edge and sometimes-unconventional health information and breakthroughs.

Referrals

Bob Lancer, the "guru of parent temper control," is an expert on child development, relationships, and team building. His many books include *Parenting with Love: Without Anger or Stress* and *Lighten Up: Harness the Power of Happiness to Create the Life You Want.*

Debbie Possehl, personal health coach, offers a clinically proven, structured, and healthy weight-loss program that works hand in hand with *Unleash the Thin Within* to ensure permanent weight loss.

Sukyo Mahikari Spiritual Development Center welcomes people from any walk of life and religion to develop their true potential as human beings.

Videos

Happy. Directed by Roko Belic. An exploration of happiness and its best predictors.

Peaceful Warrior. Adapted from Dan Millman's best-selling novel and directed by Victor Salva. A young athlete who experiences a devastating injury learns how to overcome incredible odds.

Websites

Body Ecology. Kick-start a healthier lifestyle for you and your family with Body Ecology's wealth of information, including gluten-free, sugar-free, casein-free, and probiotic-rich recipes.

Virtual Weight Loss Mirror. Discover how you will look once you reach your weight-loss goal, along with other beauty tips.

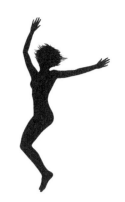

Bibliography

Introduction

American Cancer Society. "Hyperthermia." Last modified August 30, 2011. http://www.cancer.org/treatment/treatmentsand sideeffects/treatmenttypes/hyperthermia.

The Philosophy

Rosenbaum, Mike. "Fastest Mile Times: The Men's Mile World Records." About.com Track & Field. Accessed June 16, 2013. http://trackandfield.about.com/od/middledistance/p/Fastest -Mile-Times-The-Mens-Mile-World-Records.htm.

Level 1: Believe, Pray, Commit

Bruns, Chrissy, Laura McFall, Marika McFall, Tiffany Persinger, and Brooks Vostal. "Great Expectations? An Investigation of Teacher Expectation Research." Paper for EDP 603 Theories of Learning. Miami University. December 6, 2000. http://www.users.muohio.edu/shermalw/edp603_group2 -f00.html.

Dossey, Larry. *Healing Words: The Power of Prayer and the Practice of Medicine.* San Francisco: HarperSanFrancisco, 1993.

———. *Prayer Is Good Medicine: How to Reap the Healing Benefits of Prayer.* San Francisco: HarperSanFrancisco, 1996.

Emoto, Masaru. *Love Thyself: The Message from Water III.* Carlsbad, CA: Hay House, 2004.

Holistic Online. "The Proof That Prayer Works." ICBS Inc. Accessed June 16, 2013. http://1stholistic.com/prayer/hol_prayer_proof.htm.

Loehr, Franklin. *The Power of Prayer on Plants.* Garden City, NY: Doubleday, 1959. Reprint, Whitefish, MT: Kessinger Publishing, 2007.

Murray, William H. *The Scottish Himalayan Expedition.* London: J. M. Dent, 1951.

North Central Regional Educational Laboratory. "High Expectations." Accessed June 16, 2013. http://www.ncrel.org/sdrs/areas/issues/students/atrisk/at6lk11.htm.

Rosenthal, Robert, and Lenore Jacobson. "Teachers' Expectancies: Determinants of Pupils' IQ Gains." *Psychological Reports* 19 (1966): 115–18. doi: 10.2466/pr0.1966.19.1.115.

Stipek, Deborah. "How Do Teachers' Expectations Affect Student Learning?" In *Motivation to Learn: Integrating Theory and Practice*, 216-21. Boston: Allyn and Bacon, 2002. http://www.education.com/reference/article/teachers-expectations-affect-learning/.

Williams, Debra. "Scientific Research of Prayer: Can the Power of Prayer Be Proven?" *Plim Report* 8, no. 4 (1999). http://www.plim.org/PrayerDeb.htm.

Level 2: **A Better Way to Eat**

Andersen, Wayne Scott. *Dr. A's Habits of Health: The Path to Permanent Weight Control and Optimal Health.* Annapolis, MD: Habits of Health Press, 2008.

Harvard Medical School. "Truth about Fats: Bad or Good" in *The Harvard Medical School Family Health Guide.* Last modified November 2007. http://www.health.harvard.edu/fhg/updates/Truth-about-fats.shtml.

Haynes, Fiona. "Good Fats, Bad Fats, Worst Fats: Figuring Out the Fats." About.com Low Fat Cooking. Accessed June 16, 2013. http://lowfatcooking.about.com/od/lowfatbasics/a/goodfatsbadfats.htm.

Mayo Clinic. "Trans Fat Is Double Trouble for Your Heart

Health." Last modified May 6, 2011. http://www.mayo
clinic.com/health/trans-fat/CL00032.

Mercola, Joseph. "The Five Absolute Worst Foods You Can
Eat." Mercola.com. October 18, 2003. http://articles.mercola
.com/sites/articles/archive/2003/10/18/worst-foods.aspx.

———. "Saturated Fat is NOT the Cause of Heart Disease."
Mercola.com. February 25, 2010. http://articles.mercola
.com/sites/articles/archive/2010/02/25/saturated-fat-is-not
-the-cause-of-heart-disease.aspx.

Taubes, Gary. *Good Calories, Bad Calories: Challenging the
Conventional Wisdom on Diet, Weight Control, and Disease.*
New York: Knopf, 2007.

Upton, Jan. "Slow Metabolism." Lifetime Fat Loss. http://www
.lifetimefatloss.com/slow-metabolism.html.

Weil, Andrew. "Fat or Carbs: Which Is Worse?" *The Blog.* Huff
Post Healthy Living. July 2, 2010. http://www.huffington
post.com/andrew-weil-md/healthy-eating_b_629422.html.

Level 3: **Gratitude Is Key**

Batmanghelidj, Fereydoon. "The Wonders of Water: Amazing
Secrets for Health and Wellness." The Water Cure. Global
Health Solutions. Accessed June 16, 2013. http:www.water
cure.com/wondersofwater.html.

Bond, Annie B. "13 Symptoms of Chronic Dehydration."
Care2. June 7, 2008. http://www.care2.com/greenliving/
13-symptoms-of-chronic-dehydration.html.

Daino, Chris. "Our Need for Water." McVitamins. Accessed June
16, 2013. http://www.mcvitamins.com/water.htm.

Diagnose-Me.com. "Dehydration." Last modified December 14,
2012. http://www:diagnose-me.com/cond/C5223.html.

Guyton, Arthur C. *Textbook of Medical Physiology.* 8th ed. Phil-
adelphia: W. B. Saunders, 1991.

Learn about Dehydration. "12 Symptoms of Chronic Dehydration." Accessed June 16, 2013. http://dehydrationsymptoms
.org/2009/13-symptoms-of-chronic-dehydration.

Mayo Clinic. "Dehydration: Symptoms." Last modified January 7, 2011. http://www.mayoclinic.com/health/dehydration/
DS00561/DSECTION=symptoms.

Vasey, Christopher. *The Water Prescription: For Health, Vitality, and Rejuvenation*. Translated by Jon E. Graham. Rochester, VT: Healing Arts Press, 2006.

Weight Loss for All. "Benefits of Drinking Water to Lose Weight." Accessed June 16, 2013. http://www.weightlossforall.com/benefits-water-drinking.htm.

Level 4: **Make Over Your Body and Mind**

Barnett, Ola, Cindy L. Miller-Perrin, and Robin D. Perrin. *Family Violence across the Lifespan: An Introduction*. Thousand Oaks, CA: Sage Publications, 2011.

Chilton, Floyd, and Laura Tucker. *Inflammation Nation: The First Clinically Proven Eating Plan to End Our Nation's Secret Epidemic*. New York: Fireside, 2005.

Kappas, John. *Success Is Not An Accident: The Mental Bank Concept*. Van Nuys, CA: Panorama Publishing, 1987.

Mayo Clinic. "Mediterranean Diet: A Heart-Healthy Eating Plan." Last modified June 14, 2013. http://www.mayoclinic.com/health/mediterranean-diet/CL00011.

National Society for the Prevention of Cruelty to Children. "Neglect: NSPCC Research Briefing." August 2012. http://www.nspcc.org.uk/inform/research/briefings/childneglect_wda48222.html.

Talbot, Michael. *The Holographic Universe: The Revolutionary Theory of Relativity*. New York: HarperCollins, 1991.

University of Maryland Medical Center. "Omega-6 Fatty Acids." Last modified June 17, 2011. www.umm.edu/altmed/articles/omega-6-000317.htm#ixzz2PRS4Z7HW.

Level 5: **Starting to Thrive**

Barnes, Broda O., and Lawrence Galton. *Hypothyroidism: The Unsuspected Illness*. Toronto, Canada: Fitzhenry & Whiteside Limited, 1976.

He, Feng J., Caryl A. Nowson, Marilyn Lucas, and Graham A. MacGregor. "Fruit and Vegetable Consumption is Related to a Reduced Risk of Coronary Heart Disease: Meta-analysis of Cohort Studies." *Journal of Human Hypertension* 21 (2007): 717–28. doi:10.1038/sj.jhh.1002212.

Hiler, Katie. "WHAM! KAPOW! The Cellular Fight Against Free Radicals." *Health Blog*. Scienceline. Arthur J. Carter Journalism Institute. January 15, 2013. http://scienceline .org/2013/01/wham-kapow-the-cellular-fight-against -free-radicals/.

House, Paul. "Top 10 Foods Highest in Potassium." Health Alicious Ness. Accessed June 16, 2013. http://www.health aliciousness.com/articles/food-sources-of-potassium.php.

Ivker, Robert S., Robert A. Anderson, and Larry Trivieri Jr. *The Self-Care Guide to Holistic Medicine: Creating Optimal Health*. New York: Jeremy P. Tarcher/Putnam, 2000.

Kellicker, Patricia. "Volunteer Vacations: The Health Benefits of Helping Others." Beth Israel Deaconess Medical Center. Last modified June 2012. http://www.bidmc.org/Your Health/HolisticHealth/TravelandHealth.aspx?Chunk ID=78992.

Mayo Clinic. "Hypothyroidism: Symptoms." Last modified December 1, 2012. http://www.mayoclinic.com/health/ hypothyroidism/DS00353/DSECTION=symptoms.

Oz, Mehmet, and Michael Roizen. "Help Others to Help Your Health: How Giving Back Affects Your Body." *Success*. Accessed June 16, 2013. http://www.success.com/articles/1152 -drs-oz-and-roizen-help-others-to-help-your-health.

Shomon, Mary. "Thyroid Testing and Diagnosis: Clinical Evaluation, Blood Tests, Imaging Tests, Biopsies, and Other Tests." About.com Thyroid Disease. Last modified October 03, 2011. http://thyroid.about.com/od/gettestedanddiagnosed/a/testdi-agnose.htm.

Thie, John, and Matthew Thie. *Touch for Health: A Practical Guide to Natural Health with Acupressure Touch*. Camarillo, CA: De Vorss & Company, 2005. Reprint, 2012.

Level 6: Time for a Fix

American Physiological Society. "Laughter Remains Good Medicine." April 17, 2009. ScienceDaily. Accessed June 16, 2013. http://www.sciencedaily.com/releases/2009/ 04/090417084115.htm.

Buchowski M. S., K. M. Majchrzak, K. Blomquist, K. Y. Chen,

D. W. Byrne, and J. A. Bachorowski. "Energy Expenditure of Genuine Laughter." *International Journal of Obesity* 31, no. 1 (2007): 131–37. PubMed.gov. doi: 10.1038/sj.ijo.0803353.

Casey, John. "The Hidden Ingredient That Can Sabotage Your Diet." MedicineNet. WebMD. Last modified January 3, 2005. http://www.medicinenet.com/script/main/art.asp?articlekey=56589.

Cousins, Norman. *Anatomy of an Illness as Perceived by the Patient: Reflections on Healing and Regeneration.* New York: W. W. Norton, 1979.

Fiore, Kristina. "Spicy Food May Boost Metabolism." MedPage Today. August 12, 2011. http://www.medpagetoday.com/PrimaryCare/DietNutrition/28015.

Griffin, Morgan R. "Give Your Body a Boost—with Laughter: Why, for Some, Laughter Is the Best Medicine." WebMD Health & Balance. Last modified April 10, 2008. http://women.webmd.com/guide/give-your-body-boost-with-laughter.

Halton, Thomas L., and Frank B. Hu. "The Effects of High Protein Diets on Thermogenesis, Satiety, and Weight Loss: A Critical Review." *Journal of the American College of Nutrition* 23, no. 5 (October 2004): 373–85. http://www.jacn.org/content/23/5/373.full.

Kovacs, Betty. "Artificial Sweeteners." Edited by William C. Shiel. MedicineNet. WebMD. Last modified December 13, 2010. http://www.medicinenet.com/artificial_sweeteners/article.htm.

Lark, Susan M. "Foods to Avoid or Limit." In *The Women's Health Companion: Self Help Nutrition Guide and Cookbook.* Berkeley, CA: Celestial Arts, 1995. HealthWorld Online. http://www.healthy.net/Health/Article/Foods_to_Avoid_or_Limit/1378/1.

McCarraher, Lucy, and Annabel Shaw. "Happiness Habits Experiment." The Real Secret. Accessed June 16, 2013. http://www.therealsecret.net/The-Experiment.html.

Mercola, Joseph. "Sugar May Be Bad But This Sweetener Is Far More Deadly." *The Blog.* HuffPost Healthy Living. February 17, 2010. http://www.huffingtonpost.com/dr-mercola/sugar-may-be-bad-but-this_b_463655.html.

Scott, Elizabeth. "The Stress Management and Health Benefits of Laughter." About.com Stress Management. Last modified April 8, 2013. http://stress.about.com/od/stresshealth/a/laughter.htm.

Smith, Melinda, Gina Kemp, and Jeanne Segal. "Laughter is the Best Medicine: The Health Benefits of Humor and Laughter." Helpguide. Last modified November 2012. http://www.helpguide.org/life/humor_laughter_health.htm.

Strykowski, Sheri. "How to Increase Your Metabolism." Fitness Tips for Life. Accessed June 16, 2013. http://www.fitnesstipsforlife.com/10-foods-to-raise-your-metabolism.html.

Sundstrom, Kelly. "Metabolism Boosting Foods." eHow. http://www.ehow.com/facts_4812907_metabolism-boosting-foods.html.

University of Maryland Medical Center. "Green Tea." Last modified October 14, 2011. http://www.umm.edu/altmed/articles/green-tea-000255.htm.

WebMD. "Calcium: Drink Yourself Skinny." 2004. WebMD Weight Loss & Diet Plans. Accessed June 16, 2013. http://www.webmd.com/diet/features/calcium-weight-loss.

———. "Green Tea Boosts Metabolism, Protects against Diseases." WebMD Weight Loss & Diet Plans. November 28. 1999. http://www.webmd.com/diet/news/19991128/green-tea-boosts-metabolism-protects-against-diseases.

Zemel M. B., J. Richards, S. Mathis, A. Milstead, L. Gebhardt, and E. Silva. "Dairy Augmentation of Total and Central Fat Loss in Obese Subjects." *International Journal of Obesity* 29, no. 4 (2005): 391–97. doi:10.1038/sj.ijo.0802880.

Level 7: Metabolism Game Changers

Bourne, R. "New Study Finds Amount of Exercise Needed for Weight Loss." Yahoo! Health. July 31, 2008. http://voices.yahoo.com/new-study-finds-amount-exercise-needed-weight-1738823.html.

Faires, Maria. "Understanding Metabolism: How to Boost Yours with Exercise." FitDay. Accessed June 16, 2013. http://www.fitday.com/fitness-articles/fitness/understanding-metabolism-how-to-boost-yours-with-exercise.html.

———. "Understanding Metabolism: What Determines Your BMR?" FitDay. Accessed June 16, 2013. http://www.fitday .com/fitness-articles/nutrition/understanding-metabolism -what-determines-your-bmr.html.

Jakicic, John M., Bess H. Marcus, Wei Lang, and Carol Janney. "Effect of Exercise on 24-Month Weight Loss Maintenance in Overweight Women." *Archives of Internal Medicine* 168, no. 14 (July 28, 2008): 1550–59. doi:10.1001/ archinte.168.14.1550.

Kovacs, Jenny Stamos. "Increase Your Metabolism: And Start Losing Fat." WebMD Weight Loss & Diet Plans. February 2007. http://www.webmd.com/diet/features/increase-your -metabolism-start-losing-fat.

Mayo Clinic. "Metabolism and Weight Loss: How You Burn Calories." Last modified October 6, 2011. http://www.mayo clinic.com/health/metabolism/WT00006.

NHS Choices. "Causes of Constipation." Last modified March 13, 2012. http://www.nhs.uk/Conditions/Constipation/Pages/ Causes.aspx.

Nilsen, Richard. "A List of Foods & Beverages That Cause Constipation." LIVESTRONG. http://www.livestrong .com/article/275772-a-list-of-foods-beverages-that-cause- constipation/Mar 18, 2011.

Patel, Sanjay R., Atul Malhotra, David P. White, Daniel J. Gottlieb, and Frank B. Hu. "Association between Reduced Sleep and Weight Gain in Women." *American Journal of Epidemiology* 164, no. 10 (2006): 947–54. doi: 10.1093/aje/kwj280.

Skarnulis. Leanna. "What's the Best Time to Exercise?" WebMD Fitness & Exercise. May 22, 2007. http://www.webmd.com/ fitness-exercise/features/whats-the-best-time-to-exercise.

Sorgen, Carol. "Want to Lose Weight? Get Some Sleep: Getting Enough Shuteye Can Help You Get Slim." MedicineNet .WebMD. Last modified February 18, 2005. http://www .medicinenet.com/script/main/art.asp?articlekey=52027.

WebMD. "The Basics of Constipation." Last modified September 24, 2012. http:www.webmd.com/digestive-disorders/ digestive-diseases-constipation.

———. "Exercise and Weight Loss." WebMD Weight Loss & Diet

Plans. Last modified June 23, 2012. http://www.webmd
.com/diet/exercise-weight-control.

Level 8: **Positively Vibrate and Model Success**

Fritscher, Lisa. "Glossophobia: Fear of Public Speaking." About.
com Phobias. Last modified January 17, 2011. http://
phobias.about.com/od/phobiaslist/a/glossophobia.htm.

Nelson, Noelle C., and Jeannine Lemare Calaba. *The Power of
Appreciation: The Key to a Vibrant Life*. Hillsboro, OR: Beyond Words Publishing, 2003.

Peale, Norman Vincent. *The Power of Positive Thinking: A Practical Guide to Mastering the Problems of Everyday Living*.
New York: Prentice-Hall, 1952. Reprint, 2011.

Level 9: **A Healthy Body Increases Motivation**

CBS News. "Chemicals in Food Can Make You Fat." February 11, 2010. http://www.cbsnews.com/2100-500165_162-
6197493.html.

Gleason, Kathy. "What Are Lean Protein and Good Carbs?"
LIVESTRONG. Last modified June 14, 2011. http://www
.livestrong.com/article/257705-what-are-lean-protein-and
-good-carbs/.

Kornblatt, Sondra. *Better Brain at Any Age: The Holistic Way
to Improve Your Memory, Reduce Stress, and Sharpen Your
Wits*. San Francisco: Conari Press, 2009.

Lieberman, Shari, and Nancy Pauling Bruning. *Dare to Lose: 4
Simple Steps to a Better Body*. New York: Avery, 2003.

Marcantel, Tina. "Adrenal Fatigue: How Stress May Be Affect-
ing Your Health." January 23, 2010. http://www.drmarcantel.
com/medical-conditions/adrenal-fatigue/.

Mayo Clinic. "Stress: Constant Stress Puts Your Health at Risk."
Last modified September 11, 2010. http://www.mayoclinic
.com/health/stress/SR00001.

National Diabetes Information Clearinghouse. "Hypoglycemia."
National Institute of Diabetes and Digestive and Kidney
Diseases. Last modified November 6, 2012. http://
diabetes.niddk.nih.gov/dm/pubs/hypoglycemia.

New Hampshire Department of Health and Human Service.

"How Much Sugar Do You Eat?: You May Be Surprised." July 2007. http://www.dhhs.nh.gov/DPHS/nhp/adults/documents/sugar.pdf.

Pick, Marcelle. "Adrenal Health." Women to Women. Last modified May 24, 2011. http://www.womentowomen.com/adrenalhealth/adrenalfatigue.aspx.

Smith, Melinda, Maya W. Paul, and Robert Segal. "Choosing Healthy Fats: Good Fats, Bad Fats, and the Power of Omega-3s." Helpguide. Last modified December 2012. http://www.helpguide.org/life/healthy_diet_fats.htm.

Thie, John, and Matthew Thie. *Touch for Health: A Practical Guide to Natural Health with Acupressure Touch.* Camarillo, CA: De Vorss & Company, 2005. Reprint, 2012.

Veracity, Dani. "Recovering from Adrenal Fatigue: How Your Body Can Overcome Chronic Stress and Feel Energized Again." Natural News Network. April 6, 2006. http://www.naturalnews.com/019339.html.

Level 10: Be Happy, Be Vibrant, Be Alive

Jegtvig, Shereen. "Weight Management: Healthful Foods Instead of a Fad Diet." About.com Nutrition. Last modified February 14, 2013. http://nutrition.about.com/od/nutrition101/a/keep itsimple.htm.

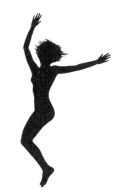

Permissions

Grateful acknowledgment is made to the following publishers and authors for permission to reprint material from their books:

Excerpts from *Love Thyself: The Message from Water III* by Marasu Emoto. Copyright © 2004 by Hay House Inc., Carlsbad, CA. Reprinted with permission of Hay House Inc.

Photographs of water crystals (pages 28 and 45) reprinted by permission of Office Marasu Emoto LLC.

Neurovascular holding points and neurolymphatic massage points (pages 68, 104–105) from the 2012 reprinting of the 2005 edition of *Touch for Health: A Practical Guide to Natural Health with Acupressure Touch* (complete edition) by John Thie and Matthew Thie, and photography by Chuck Behrman. ISBN 9780875168715. Reprinted with permission of DeVorss Publications.

Commitment passage (page 31) from *The Scottish Himalayan Expedition* by William H. Murray. Published by the Orion Publishing Group. First published 1951 by J. M. Dent. All attempts at tracing the copyright holder of *The Scottish Himalayan Expedition* were unsuccessful.

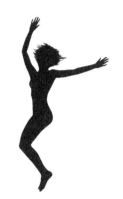

Photo Credits

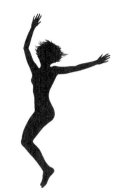

About the Author

MARGIANNA LANGSTON is a trainer, speaker, and professional manager with formidable experience teaching and motivating people in nonprofit, corporate, and government environments.

As the director of Disaster Preparedness and Recovery for United Way of Metropolitan Atlanta, Margianna led disaster recovery efforts for more than two hundred organizations. She and her team were instrumental in providing relief for the victims of the 2009 Atlanta floods, the Haiti earthquake medical evacuees and caregivers, and the 100,000 victims of Hurricane Katrina who evacuated to Atlanta.

As a nutritional consultant, Ms. Langston set up a preventive-medicine department in a local physician's general practice and counseled patients. She is also a certified neuro-linguistic professional with the Robbins Research Institute and has taught *Mental Bank: Success Is Not an Accident* in the Atlanta area.

Margianna holds two bachelor of science degrees, one in business with a focus on marketing and the other in nutrition.

She has received several notable community service honors, including an award from WSB Radio for her work with local nonprofit organizations. Ms. Langston lives in Decatur, Georgia.

CPSIA information can be obtained at www.ICGtesting.com
Printed in the USA
LVOW02s0747190713

343638LV00002B/2/P